Medical Education, Accreditation and the Nation's Health: Reflections of an Atypical Dean

Medical Education, Accreditation
and
the Nation's Health

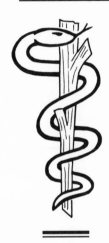

Reflections
of an
Atypical Dean

by Andrew D. Hunt

Michigan State University Press
East Lansing, Michigan
1991

Michigan State University Press
East Lansing, Michigan 48823-5202
Copyright © 1990 Andrew D. Hunt

All Michigan State University Press books are produced
on paper which meets the requirements of American
National Standard for Information Sciences—
Permanence of paper for printed materials. ANSI 239.48–
1984.

Printed in the United States of America

Library of Congress Cataloging-in-Publication Data

Hunt, Andrew D.
    Medical education, accreditation, and the nation's
    health: reflections of an atypical dean / Andrew D.
    Hunt.
        p. cm.
    Includes index.
    ISBN 0-87013-288-1
    1. Medical education—United States. 2. Physicians—
    Certification—United States. 3. Medical care—United
    States.
    I. Title.
    R745.H86   1991
    610'.71173—dc20   90-50845
                                                  CIP

0

To my four children: George, Holly, Judy, and Robin, who were totally supportive of the multiple moves and dislocations which are part and parcel of my nomadic career, and to my devoted wife, Lotta, who was always there.

Contents

Acknowledgments

This volume was partially prepared while the author was a fellow at the Center for Advanced Study in the Behavioral Sciences. I am grateful for finacial support provided by the Henry J. Kaiser Family Foundation. The author is indebted for help provided by the William T. Grant Foundation for travel in preparation of this volume.

I give special thanks to Peter O. Ways, M.D., personal friend and vital contributor to our college at Michigan State, who painstakingly read, criticized, and made many recommindations for an early version of the manuscript that significantly shaped its final form.

1
Introduction

This book is about medicine and health care in the United States, with special emphasis on the education of physicians. The academic medical center, where physicians and most other health professionals are educated and trained for clinical practice and from which most of their life-long post-graduate education stems, holds the central position of this system. It is the model for ambitious community hospitals. The academic medical center, indeed, is a dominant force in the way health care is provided for the public. Any significant changes in the health care system can be expected only with appropriate responses and leadership by the academic establishment. This idea will be developed from the base of historical narrative, and will be correlated with my own experiences when such intrusion of personal observations seems justified.

While this monograph is not intended to be autobiographical, my life work has taken me into the mainstream of medical education in a continuing effort to be in the forefront of change. Thus, while I have enjoyed some success, and have become generally accepted in this role, conflict with educational traditionalists and the medical school accreditation establishment has been an inevitable byproduct of my prickly personality and change-oriented style. Although many of these disagreements have been frustrating, my insights into the shortcomings of the health care system and the degree to which medical education is responsible for the perpetuation of these problems have been sharpened.

I am seventy-four years old, and in semi-retirement from a career spent almost entirely in the field of medical education that reached its peak in 1964 when I became founding dean of the new medical school at Michigan State University. I am now a part-time associate dean at Mercer University School of Medicine, also a new institution dedicated to an innovative curriculum designed to promote interest in primary care in rural Georgia. Both schools deliberately assumed the need for pedagogical and organizational innovation in order to promote their goals of community service and scientific productivity. Especially in their earliest developmental periods, this brought

1

them into considerable conflict with the academic establishment through struggles with the accreditation process, that inevitably reflected the attitudes of the power structure of their parent organizations—the American Medical Association (AMA) and the Association of American Medical Colleges (AAMC).

I now spend each academic year in a resort community in the Southeast that adjoins an industrial town of about 16,000. Its 350-bed community hospital and its specialty-oriented medical staff of about 130 physicians provide medical care for the community's population and act as a referral center for a large rural area. A number of these physicians hold clinical appointments at Mercer—200 miles away—and serve both as preceptors for medical students in the four-year rural practitioner-based preceptorship program, and as teachers in specialty-based elective clerkships for senior students.

Referral centers, to which these physicians send most of their more complex cases, are located in two larger communities, each about ninety minutes away. The local hospital, sometimes in collaboration with Mercer, maintains an active program in continuing medical education that is organized and coordinated by a hospital-based pathologist who also works closely with Mercer in its program of medical student rotations. The physicians who serve as voluntary preceptors are highly rated by the students, and hospital personnel, without house staff, has come to enjoy their leavening presence. The hospital staff is ambitious for the institution, has developed a cardiac catheterization program with a cardiac team from one of the referral hospitals, and looks forward to the day when such tertiary procedures as cardiac surgery will be done here.

Two years ago, I experienced a major encounter with the medical system. I elaborate here because the story illustrates American community-based medicine at its very best, the excellence of tertiary care in a modern community hospital, and the availability of well trained specialists in cities not endowed with academic medical centers. It also reveals certain shortcomings in the conduct of hospital patient care and in the organization of private medical practice which does not always work to the patient's best interest. The cost of the procedure also stands as stark evidence to explain why this kind of medical care is decreasingly available to the poor and uninsured. It is my belief that these deficiencies, due to multiple causes, can in large part be traced to serious gaps in the scope of medical education and to the current role of the academic medical center in modern society. The experience buttresses my belief that successful modification of our system, supported by physicians and other health professionals, can occur only through leadership from both organized medicine and the medical education establishment.

In the first place, my experience demonstrates the value of the periodic health checkup, and the importance of good doctor-patient communication, understanding, and trust. During the previous

2

couple of years I had noticed increasing memory difficulties and possible facial asymmetry while smiling, but otherwise no apparently relevant symptoms. I had taken this in stride, feeling that it was all a normal inconvenience of aging but, somewhat sheepishly, reported this turn of events to my internist during my annual check-up. He was wisely skeptical of the "aging" hypothesis, and I was sent to radiology for a CAT scan. This procedure revealed an orange-sized well-circumscribed tumor that occupied a large part of the space normally reserved for the left brain. Immediate surgical intervention was clearly demanded. A stranger to the neurosurgical resources in this part of the country, I relied on his judgment, which was in favor of a neurological group 60 miles away instead of the academic medical center 250 miles distant. He felt that the combination of surgical skill and hospital competency was equal to that of the university hospital, and that we would all be better served closer to home. I was suddenly a medical emergency, being referred to a totally strange hospital and surgeon for what clearly was to be a serious, and possibly risky, procedure. The confidence that my wife and I had for our primary care physician, however, diminished our anxiety.

The hospitalization experience was a revelation that provided me not only with a first-hand understanding of what it is like to be really ill, but also clarified some issues involved in community hospitals providing tertiary care. My hospitalization, originally estimated at ten days or so, turned out to be a month. In addition to the initial eight hours in the operating room, I returned within forty-eight hours because of hemorrhage at the tumor site, and again within a week to insert a drain to relieve built-up air pressure. However, in spite of three extensive surgical interventions, the results have been spectacular. I never had more than a mild headache, and from the beginning of the post-operative course the speech therapist could find no evidence of impairment. Twenty months later I am totally free of the memory problems and the facial asymmetry which, in retrospect, had been real symptoms and signs.

The 350-bed hospital is beautifully equipped for post-operative neurosurgical intensive care, and the nursing staff is adept in complexities of ministering to patients in this setting. They know the equipment, are skilled in starting and maintaining intravenous fluids and, in general, were a self-sufficient team that inspired my confidence as a patient. The hospital is well-supplied with state-of-the-art diagnostic equipment, and with highly professional technicians who were courteous and sensitive in applying their technology to the typically uncomfortable and demanding post-operative patient.

In many respects, then, the academic medical center had been reproduced in this community setting. The surgical expertise, furnishings, and relevant equipment equaled that of most distinguished university hospitals; indeed, they were possibly better, for university hospitals periodically suffer financial setbacks that seem less likely to occur in modern and ambitious community hospitals. Furthermore, specialty residents, who are learning their trade, may well do much of the actual surgery in the university setting. While this works in the patients' best interests in the long run, inexperience can generate problems in individual situations. The patient under the care of a qualified surgeon in private practice in a hospital with no house staff need not worry about such an eventuality.

While the physical structure of this hospital closely simulated an academic medical center, it differed strikingly in medical staffing pattern. In the academic medical center, the responsible physicians are usually fulltime and are based in either the hospital or the adjacent medical school. When "on service," these physicians are responsible for a group of patients who are, in fact, their primary concern. Furthermore, house staff on service have responsibility for first-call attention on the basis of a very short response time. Thus, if the academic system is working properly, a hospitalized patient in need should have an intern or resident at his side within minutes, with the ward chief, if needed, not far behind. While house staff's primary purpose of being trained may at times threaten the best technical surgical procedure, their presence as medical care givers is a special feature of the academic institution.

The primary medical responsibility for hospitalized patients in the community setting is the private practicing physician, whose office is usually outside the hospital, who may have several hospital appointments, and whose attention must inevitably be distracted from the immediate needs of hospitalized patients by a filled waiting room. In the absence of a house staff, the general method of coping is for practicing physicians to make scheduled hospital rounds once or twice daily. Needs of hospitalized patients may be dealt with through telephoned instructions to floor nurses, by dispatching someone such as a "physicians' assistant" to check out the situation, or the physician may simply leave the office to the dismay of those awaiting attention there. In any case, the surgeon or other specialist whose patients are susceptible to crises must constantly deal with the dilemma of where to direct attention.

My postoperative course was adversely affected by this system. In this institution nurses did some of the routine checking that was normally the responsibility of physicians or was assigned to house staff, where present. Thus, although they listened to my chest daily, most of them seemed to lack appropriate skill, the development of which is not normally included in education for nursing. For whatever reason, the early signs of my approaching crisis were missed for several days, by which time I had spiked a fever, was coughing, and had become seriously ill. When the pulmonologist was finally called he discovered that I had suffered a pulmonary embolism. Furthermore, I feel certain that it was only at the insistence of my

4

wife, who was trained in nursing, that my need for immediate specialized medical attention was noted.

The other major problem in my hospitalization had to do with nutrition, a problem that applies to most hospitals, teaching or community. I lost twenty-five pounds during my hospitalization. On discharge, I was weak, emaciated, and essentially unable to walk; indeed, suffering from moderate malnutrition. Some of such weight loss can be attributed to the inevitable systemic impact of surgery, anesthesia, and complex postoperative metabolic changes. I attribute it more however to the administrative custom of separating patient feeding from medical and nursing control, and placing this activity within a semi-autonomous department generally called "food service." This system may well work for the patient for whom the act of eating is not a problem, but it failed miserably for me. Soon after coming out of anesthesia, I was put on a "regular" diet and asked to choose from a menu with such options as pork chops or fried chicken. Eating food of that kind was impossible, even with my wife feeding me. I should have been offered soft or liquid foods such as milk shakes during these first days of the postoperative period, with the gradual introduction of solids carefully chosen for their specific nutritional value. Nutrition should have been part of the medical-nursing postoperative plan. Physicians and medical educators are frequently criticized for their insouciance about nutrition as reflected in these kinds of situations, in which medical attention is largely limited to the specialized problem at hand, rather than to the patient's total needs.

I have not yet computed the total cost of this procedure and hospitalization. As a "senior citizen" I have Medicare coverage, and an additional private insurance policy which generally fills the gap between the actual billing and the Medicare payment. The total hospital bill for this month of care was a little over $45,000. A large portion of this bill was for high-technology tests and procedures which were essential for accuracy in diagnosis and effectiveness of treatment. I learned from this experience the enormous benefits to patients of, for example, the CAT scan and magnetic resonance imaging (MRI), which combined to replace the painful air encephalogram—which had been "de rigeur" in my residency days, and which caused such misery to brain tumor patients as spinal fluid was removed and air was injected to delineate the shape and location of a tumor on x-ray film. Furthermore, it is important for such resources to be reasonably available to patients, rather than limited to large referral centers. The issue is clearly not the existence or validity of such technology, but the need for strategies to make it available and affordable for the population at large.

In my case, there was never any discussion with my physicians of fees, although I was assured that they would be covered by my combined insurance protection. Indeed, my mail has been loaded

5

with copies of Medicare worksheets, handled in this state through a private insurance firm. These have revealed, in addition to the neurosurgeon's fee, those of two sets of radiologists, a cardiologist for the interpretation of an electrocardiogram, an anesthesiologist, laboratory pathologists, and a pulmonologist. So far, I have in my file about forty such statements. This must represent several hundred dollars in clerical and secretarial help, postage, and office supplies paid from public funds in support of the current fee-for-service style of private medical practice. This has also been an inconvenience for me, for a number of local and long-distance phone calls, as well as letters requesting information have been necessary to keep the whole billing process straight. With all its difficulties, however, Medicare, combined with an unusually effective private insurance company, have managed to cover the costs of my illness, not only for the hospital, but for the services of all the physicians involved.

In spite of the complications I experienced, the system worked well for me, a semi-retired physician living comfortably in a resort community, and enjoying the deference with which medical professionals care for each other. Indeed, my hospital experience, notwithstanding its complications, epitomizes the pinnacle of the American health care system, and falls into the same general category as transplantation, open-heart surgery, intensive care, and the whole gamut of illnesses and conditions responsive to high-technology medical and surgical care. Such medical diversity is now found throughout the country, with much of the needed technology and specialized personnel located not only in academic medical centers but in many medium-sized communities that support specialists and hospitals such as the one in which I received my care. The entire system, generally working within the paradigm of private enterprise, and fueled and intellectually dominated by medical schools and their academic medical centers, has clearly worked wonders and justifies its distinction as the "greatest health care in the world."

The purpose of this monograph, however, is not to dwell on our successes, but rather to analyze the problems that may threaten the very existence of medicine as we now define it. My own neurosurgical experience, while surely a success, reveals problems of tertiary hospital care in community settings. Community programs in areas of tertiary care such as neurosurgery, intensive care, neonatology, and cardiovascular surgery need to find ways to insure the best possible in-hospital care by supplementing the practicing physician with some degree of hospital-based medical support. Strategies for insuring prompt physician response time include the hospital as primary locus for referring medical specialists' offices, and the management of the community-based private office in such a way as to insure the presence of an appropriately informed and skilled physician within the hospital at all times. The family practice residency, as a program available to the community hospital, is an option sometimes open to hospital management. While not expected to provide the specialized kind of care available in the academic medical center, such residents are quite capable of identifying postsurgical complications and other unexpected emergencies indigenous to the hospital. Finally, if such traditionally medical responsibility is to be vested with nurses or other nonphysician professionals, it is incumbent on the hospital staff and administration to set up relevant training programs to insure their necessary competence.

By and large, my case history is metaphor for the very best side of American medicine. It demonstrates the remarkable capacity of this service-oriented version of private enterprise to educate physicians, train specialists, get them started in the small business of private office practice, and become effective members of the medical-industrial complex. They are aided in getting set up by drug companies, office equipment and furniture manufacturers, and banks from which they obtain favorable loans so that within relatively few years they are doing well financially and are providing a high level of medical care to those who can afford their services. As a group, they are conscientious, attend their specialty meetings for continuing education, and regularly read relevant medical journals. Many participate in various educational programs for medical students if they are located near medical schools. In short, it is hard to fault their professional function, although the physician's capacity to discipline or regulate his fellows is generally not outstanding.

The distribution of medical care in this country, like housing and other products and services in the private sector, is designed for a middle- and upper-class clientele which, either directly out of earnings or through a plethora of health insurance programs, can pay for services rendered. Like any private sector entrepreneur, the practicing physician must be continually conscious of the bottom line, and resents having more than a modicum of patients who do not somehow pay their way. Thus, entitlements such as Medicaid, which usually pay considerably less than the amount the physician has established as an appropriate fee, are unpopular, and some physicians tend to exclude patients so financed from their practices. In this day of high office expenses and the ubiquitous anxiety about malpractice and its increasing cost of insurance, the physician is indeed restricted in the volume of services he can deliver on a charitable basis.

Community hospitals, whether under the aegis of cities or counties, whether designated "non-profit" institutions, units of "for-profit" hospital corporations, or "non-profit" hospitals with management contracts with "for-profit" chains, are in the same bind as are practicing physicians. Geared for "breaking even" or for showing a profit, ever-increasing costs of operation force rates to be frequently raised; the burden of caring for non-paying, or even part-paying patients must be kept to a minimum. While it may be the

7

case that needy patients when severely ill or injured are rarely refused hospital care, the financial burden imposed by them is difficult to manage; and the periodic tendency for Medicaid and Medicare to reduce payments to hospitals is further cause for concern.

A recent addition to the many ways in which the poor find participation in the medical care system difficult is the transfer of some essential elements of good preventive medicine from city or county health departments to private hospitals and physicians' offices. While physicians have always given immunizations, provided dietary advice, and run no-smoking sessions, the community's poor have generally used the local health department as the affordable source of these same services. Now, however, organizations such as national and regional cancer societies are proclaiming the essential nature of such procedures as annual mammograms and biannual colonoscopies in nationally oriented programs such as the "war against cancer." These examinations are generally available only in physicians' offices or hospitals, and are often not covered by existing governmental entitlements. Even if a health department or community-oriented clinic wanted to provide such preventive medical services, the cost would be prohibitive without burdensome cost sharing by its medically indigent patients.

The American health care system, then, composed of medical private practice, hospitals, pharmaceutical houses, equipment manufacturers, insurance companies, and other related agencies, is a medical-industrial complex that has been extraordinarily effective in providing care to much of the middle- and upper-class populations. Medical schools and their academic medical centers, with research programs funded largely from the National Institutes of Health, are an essential and driving force within the complex. They are not only the source of most of the nation's physicians, but are also the resource through which the vast majority of physicians' lifelong continuing education and acculturation is provided. They originate new parameters of care, generate most of the new medically-oriented technology and, with their ever-increasing emphasis on highly specialized tertiary care, have become a sort of template for nonacademic hospitals throughout the nation.

While the system tends to serve the middle and upper classes well, with its steeply escalating cost still barely falling within the scope of most health insurance plans, there is clear danger that it could price itself out of the market. This has already occurred, for example, in the case of Medicaid, whose payments are failing to meet costs in either physicians' offices or hospitals. With the poor apparently increasing in number, with an increasing tendency toward parttime employment to absolve employers of the need to provide health insurance, and with the ominous implications of dangerous epidemics of AIDS and Alzheimer's disease, collapse of the system seems far from impossible.

The ways in which the problem of costs will ultimately be

resolved is not yet clear. We have recently seen a dramatic decline of international enthusiasm for governmentally managed socialistic economies, and of strengthened American antipathy to socialistic solutions for our own economic and social problems. With free enterprise as political philosophy stronger than ever, and in view of the likelihood of continuation of conservative politics in the United States, a major shift of the locus of health care to the public sector seems unlikely. Somehow, at least for the foreseeable future, we must make do with the medical industrial complex essentially as it is, capitalize on its strengths, and explore ways in which it can work with the public sector to achieve some measure of justice to insure accessibility to all segments of our population. Modifications of this system, some suggested by my personal case history, are needed to uplift its potential for uniformly excellent patient care. The more urgent changes, however, must occur within the political and economic domains of human activity, and concern themselves with ways in which, generally available, high-quality health care can emerge from the currently restricted and stratified health-oriented entitlements which, already inadequate, can become political footballs for the resolution of unrelated national issues. An intensively collaborative effort between the public and private sectors will be needed and will require a heretofor rare level of physician cooperation and support. This monograph will not consider the content of the various current plans; rather, it will dwell upon the critical nature of medical education in preparing physicians for effective participation in this process.

Whatever plan does materialize, its true effectiveness can only be realized with the cooperation of a medical profession oriented around the need for such a development, that participates actively in the planning, and that is prepared for significant modifications in ways of doing business. Such an orientation for a profession that is, fundamentally, politically, and fiscally conservative, is not likely to emerge spontaneously. Unless a struggle the dimensions of that which accompanied the advent of Medicare in the early 1960s were to be repeated, a large-scale infusion of information and revision of attitudinal and problem-solving paradigms would be a necessary condition for the wholehearted involvement of physicians and their professional and commercial colleagues in the complex and difficult process needed for a successful outcome.

The source of this enormous educational effort would have to be the physicians' national professional organizations, namely, the American Medical Association and the Association of American Medical Colleges. The AMA, through its Council on Medical Education and Hospitals, and its joint participation in medical school accreditation through the Liaison Committee for Medical Education (LCME), has historically been supportive of medical education. It has recently seemed somewhat more inclined toward emphasis on primary care and other socially-relevant issues than have most traditional medical schools, or even the AAMC itself. However, its basic function as the central agency of the practicing medical community has perforce focused much of its energy on representing and promoting the interests of practitioners and their constituent (county) medical societies, and it would probably be unreasonable to expect it to take leadership in attempting to effect major behavioral or attitudinal change on behalf of its membership.

The main responsibility for initiating and sustaining such a mammoth program would belong to the AAMC. There is every reason to believe that the AMA and its constituent societies could become effective partners in that effort. Indeed, through speeches at plenary sessions by deans, association presidents, and invited speakers, AAMC annual meetings have characteristically enjoined medical schools to pioneer in venturesome innovations in curriculum and demonstration programs. However, the association's power structure, concerned as it must be with issues of financing its schools, maintaining increasing extramural research funding, and promoting continued viability of university hospitals, tends to find such departures from tradition at best a secondary priority to the more insistent and seemingly life-or-death issues of daily academic existence. The traditionalistic force reveals itself throughout the academic system, and includes accreditation decisions, criteria for faculty appointment and promotion, curriculum content, and values expressed in the selection of those members of the academic community for special distinction through lectureships and awards.

Political action by the AAMC, largely at the federal level, has been concentrated around maintenance of the funding and scientific health of the NIH and, at times, around specific graduate programs and special educational projects. Rarely, if ever, has it paid particular attention to issues of public funding for medical care, except insofar as it affects reimbursement for university hospitals and medical faculty for the care of publicly funded patients. Clearly, these priorities would have to change were true leadership toward improved public funding for medical care to become a major preoccupation of academic medicine. This monograph, through historical analysis, will attempt to identify reasons for the current position of academic medicine, and to suggest ways in which it might be transformed into an effective agent for national change.

In addition to change in public funding for medical care, there is also need for modifying the way medical care is organized at the community level. My own case history has revealed the general capability of modern and aggressive community hospitals and their specialized staffs to cope with serious medical and surgical problems. I reemphasize, however, that top-notch care of hospitalized patients requires faster response times than can be provided by physicians who, no matter how dedicated, must simultaneously attend to office-based practices outside the hospital. Some sort of full-time hospital-based and suitably trained professional must be

10

available, whether in the form of house staff, practicing physicians doing fulltime periodic duty or, as is the case in most of Europe, hospital-based specialists who are limited to referral practice. Early in the 1950s, the American equivalent of a modified European arrangement was demonstrated as a health care experiment in a rural New Jersey county where I was director of pediatric services.[1] While this particular arrangement has never been exactly duplicated, we demonstrated that capable specialists could function as fulltime chiefs of service without threatening the autonomy or scope of primary care practitioners, and that the quality of such hospital care could be of the highest order. While such demonstrations of communitywide innovation in the provision of medical care deserve support, recognition, and encouragement from the AMA and AAMC, they are fundamentally the fruits of local initiative. The Hunterdon experiment evolved from the enlightened leadership of influential citizens who wanted first class medical care for their semirural county. They sought academic and foundation consultation, funding, and affiliation, and became a powerful and effective board of trustees.

I think it is important for community hospital boards and ambitious medical staffs to realize that in duplicating the activities of the academic medical center at the community level, the presence of qualified technically skilled surgeons, state-of-the-art hospital equipment, and well-trained nurses and technicians are only part of what is necessary. While the degree to which a community hospital may wish to involve itself in relevant training programs will depend on the local situation, the effectiveness with which patients get prompt, efficient, and humane care must be of universal concern. This is an administrative as well as a professional matter.

While the Hunterdon experience revealed that such an arrangement was feasible within the paradigm of private enterprise medicine, the traditional status of the practicing specialist as an independent practitioner managing both office and hospital practices was modified so that the needs of the hospital patient were met by a hospital-based group of salaried specialists who were initially supported by a foundation grant, and ultimately through fees-for-service. As chief of pediatrics, I was responsible for the care of newborn infants and hospitalized children. While most patients continued to be under the care of their family physicians, I made daily rounds, discussed problems with the attending doctors, suggested modifications in diagnostic or treatment modalities, responded to most emergency situations, and submitted appropriate bills for my services. Usually, when the illness was really severe (poliomyelitis was epidemic), the patient was officially turned over to me. Along with others in the specialist group, I saw patients in a hospital office, mostly on referral from the practitioner-staff members. By and large, the arrangement worked well, and after my departure, continued in this fashion under an able successor.[2]

11

A great peril faced by the health care system, even within the context of its basic service objectives toward the paying public, is its ever-inflating cost. This area has attracted attention at all levels and cost containment, in one form or another, is an objective in most medical curricula. Nonetheless, at the community level, when physicians and hospitals know their bills will be paid, concern for costs is rarely of paramount concern. For example, in my case, the brain tumor had been clearly diagnosed by a well-executed CAT scan in our community hospital on Monday; on Thursday, even though I had taken the original films with me, the first thing done was to repeat this $500 test at the new hospital. This duplication was probably unnecessary, and is an example of inadvertent profligacy whose continued practice is incompatible with long-term solvency of the system. It is my feeling that this tendency is a continuance of what I call the "grand-rounds syndrome," in honor of that epitome of medical school teaching performance—departmental grand rounds. In this weekly disease-oriented exercise, the professor tends to cover all diagnostic parameters relating to possible etiology or relevance to understanding of basic scientific principles, regardless of their importance to the patient's actual diagnosis or therapeutic needs. All tests must be displayed on slides or on charts, and preferably under the aegis of the school's own consultants and laboratories. This kind of performance has been the main manifestation of the supreme academic role model and, I believe, strongly influences medical graduates throughout their lives.

Indeed, due to medical practice styles and the intrinsic price of modern medical interventions, the 15 percent inflation rate of medical care consistently outpaces that of the general economy. The current 12 percent of the gross national product going to the health establishment is generally considered to be exorbitant and incompatible with the nation's fiscal well-being. While those of us who are well-covered by adequate health insurance have thus far been able to cope with this cost escalation, we too are now threatened by the beginning flight from the health field by insurance companies. For example, TIAA-CREF, the largest corporation providing retirement income for American academics, is currently abandoning its major-medical coverage, and Blue Cross premiums across the nation are escalating almost beyond the level of tolerance. There is real urgency for physicians to use the laboratory and costly procedures sparingly, only in the patient's best interests and with due regard for his autonomy and right to accept or reject proffered medical ministrations. Whether or not the procedure or test is covered by insurance should rarely be a factor in medical decision-making. Such issues should be an extensive part of the content of formal medical education, both at the undergraduate and graduate levels, should be displayed in the faculty's demonstration of ideal patient care, and should be included in the context of continuing education.

12

By far the most sinister flaw in the system, however, is its relative inaccessibility by much of this country's disadvantaged population. There seem to be over 35 million uninsured people. While the elderly are covered by Medicare, and certain eligible categories of the poor qualify for Medicaid support, there are serious gaps in each of these programs. The Medicare program for seniors is in jeopardy because of the current press to utilize all governmental funds for deficit reduction at the expense of eligible recipients, and by the resentment with which some methods for physician and hospital reimbursement have been received. This dissonance results in part from attempts to contain costs through various efforts to put ceilings on hospital and physician charges. Medicaid, a program shared by state and federal governments, varies greatly in effectiveness and equity. Even were these two programs to work to the satisfaction of all concerned, many categories of poor people would still not be covered. There is, for example, an increasing number of minimum-wage level employees, particularly in service industries, who are hired on a parttime status partly to relieve employers from providing required health insurance. Such individuals, particularly if formerly accustomed to union-provided health insurance, find themselves suddenly among the medically indigent.

The theme of this introduction has been to suggest that all aspects of the changes needed to perfect the delivery of medical care to the segment of the public which pays its own way, and to extend those benefits to recipients who are now either partly franchised or not franchised at all, will require the intense cooperation and involvement of the medical profession—not only in its own performance but also in an unaccustomed spirit of collaboration with state and federal governments.

The academic establishment has provided good leadership in the application of research findings and engineering developments to medical care, and the diffusion of such information to the profession has been highly effective. While we will see later that some medical schools have made moves to expand the notion of physician responsibility beyond that which can be encompassed within the purview of biomedicine, we will also discover that the rich history of the centrality of research in the educational value system, together with the insistent application of these standards to the medical school accreditation process, has often served as a deterrent to serious innovation relevant to the problems of medicine and society.

This historically-based narrative will proceed in the following sequence. In chapter 2 we will consider the history of modern medical education, the way in which it was reformed at turn of this century, adopted the German tradition of university standards of excellence, and accepted the German idea of research as the center of and highest value in professorial performance and educational importance. We will proceed to consider modern times, with the Association of American Medical Colleges, its historic relationship to the AMA, and it guiding forces and their ambivalence vis-à-vis continued research supremacy and broader educational philosophies.

The issues of educational reform as it has proceeded in American medical schools since the mid-1950s, the growth of research in medical education as a field of endeavor, and the degree to which it has been encouraged by the AAMC will be considered in chapter 3. The addition of behavioral and social scientists to the faculties of some medical schools, and the growth of medical humanities—particularly medical ethics—as highly relevant areas of scholarship for faculty and medical students, will be described. Family practice, as a new primary care specialty, will be discussed, along with its potential importance as issues of primary care, rural medicine, and accessibility of medical care to vulnerable population groups become areas of academic interest.

In chapter 4 we will deal with the extramural support system for medical schools, particularly for research. The vital role of charitable foundations as they contributed to research itself and to various other aspects of support for medical education during the first half of the century will be discussed. The main emphasis will be on the post-World War II development of federal support systems for research, especially the National Institutes of Health. The phenomenal growth of this system, and the uniquely American combination of political and organized laymen's energy in its original establishment, will be described. Finally, we will consider the impact of this new-found source of research and research-training support on the medical schools resulting in a metamorphosis to their current status as imposing and complex research and tertiary care institutes within which education of physicians, nurses, graduate students, and other related health personnel occurs almost as byproducts of the main institutional goal—the advancement of scientific medicine. The implications of this sequence of events will be discussed.

The history and locus of the accreditation mechanism for medical schools will be treated in chapter 5. These will be traced from the original initiatives of the AMA, the adoption of the process by the AAMC, and their eventual fusion within the current context of the Liaison Committee on Medical Education. Areas of tension, such as that between the LCME and the various regional accreditation bodies for higher education in general, and between its self-accreditation features and the antitrust aspects of federal law, will be discussed. While the process has been effective in guaranteeing the flow of well-trained physicians, the basically conservative position of biomedical research has been a major factor in inhibiting the accreditation process from encouraging imaginative innovative development, particularly within some of the new medical schools that have emerged during the past three decades. I will illustrate this inhibitory process in my narrative about the two new schools with which I have been involved. I will conclude with the observation that there may be some change taking place in the membership of the LCME and that, with new personnel at the staff level at the AAMC and AMA, there could soon be alternatives in criteria for successful accreditation, and assumption of leadership by accreditation in effecting desirable and important change in medical education.

In chapter 6, a summary of this monograph, I will attempt to set out a rational hypothetical agenda for American medical education should it decide to undertake the leadership role in transformation of American medicine which I think appropriate. Paramount would be a need to support the idea that revision of some of the current bench-research oriented ideology of medicine must be supplemented with an equally powerful humanistic and social component in order for medicine to continue to thrive in its productive position in the private enterprise system, and to serve the nation with maximum effectiveness.

NOTES

1. R. E. Trussel, *Hunterdon Medical Center: The Story of One Approach to Rural Medical Care* (Cambridge: Harvard University Press, 1956).
2. A. J. Bambara, A. D. Hunt, Jr., "Specialist Plus, Not Versus, Family Physician: A Setting Conducive to Effective Postgraduate Education," *Postgraduate Medicine* 20 (1956): 305–9; and A. D. Hunt, Jr., "At a Rural Hospital" (part of a symposium on the hospitalized child), *Children* 3 (1956): 90.

2
The AAMC and Its Relationship to the AMA

The national organization that serves and monitors medical schools of the United States and Canada is the Association of American Medical Colleges (AAMC). Its membership includes deans, faculty, and students of medical schools, and teaching hospitals. While its major event, the annual meeting, is attended by thousands of members, it is a functional organization, located in Washington, D.C. It works closely with the federal government, develops positions on issues relevant to the needs and conditions of medical schools, keeps records on many aspects of medical education, shares responsibility for medical school accreditation with the American Medical Association (AMA) and, in general, serves as an umbrella organization. Its staff is divided into such departments as the Office of the President, Government Relations, Administrative Services, Computer Services, Communications, Biomedical Research, Academic Affairs, Institutional Planning and Development, and Clinical Services. Its budget for 1986–87 was a little over $13 million, with assets totaling more than $22 million.

My first experience at an AAMC annual meeting was in 1964 after I had become dean of the fledgling College of Human Medicine at Michigan State University. I had accepted this task largely because of the encouragement of Dr. Ward Darley, then executive director of the AAMC. Under his leadership, the AAMC had been actively encouraging a change of emphasis in medical education through such efforts as sponsoring a series of teaching institutes. (This will be treated in more detail in chapter 3. See notes 11-18 for that chapter.) At that meeting he expressed delight that I had accepted a position which showed so much promise for administrative and curricular innovation in support of the educational research that had been encouraged by his organization. As I later discovered, the accrediting body found many of the very administrative and pedagogical innovations that we felt appropriate to Michigan State to be more than the visiting teams and the parent body could accept.

17

This organizational ambivalence—liberal and explorative at the level of administrative leadership, but traditional and loath to risk change at the level of the true power structure—has seemed throughout my academic life to be a prominent organizational characteristic.

The AAMC, still relatively small and often characterized as a "dean's club" during Ward Darley's tenure as executive director, decided that it needed to expand and enlarge its representation in the universities and their medical schools and to promote more effectiveness in its relationship with government. A committee, chaired by Lowell Coggeshall, earlier president of the University of Washington, was appointed to develop appropriate recommendations for this new scope of the AAMC.[1] (Details of this report will be described later in this chapter.)

The AAMC now (in 1990), has become a huge, complex organization essential for the successful function of its member medical schools with their ever increasing problems and complexity. This, and the administrative demands placed on the staff by such diverse activities, may have diluted the emphasis on educational issues so prominent before expansion. The earlier history of the AAMC needs to be understood, however, in order to evaluate the post-1965 changes.

EARLY HISTORY

The early history of the AAMC, while identifiable as a separate story, is in fact closely interwoven with that of other groups—namely the AMA, licensing boards, relevant foundations, and selected universities. This history is complex and has been studied and narrated by numerous authors, [2] and the current account will be brief. The details, however, are intended to provide a background explanation of the current attitudes and activities of this organization which has done so much to catalyze the development of today's system of medical education and health care.

The history of the AAMC prior to about 1960 has not been extensively documented; hence, I have borrowed heavily from an informative and well written paper by Smiley.[3] The founding of the AAMC in May 1876, and the content of that first meeting in Philadelphia as well as the election of J. B. Biddle, M.D., of Jefferson Medical College as the first president, is described. Twenty-two medical colleges were represented and actions which suggested the need for drastic improvement in medical education were taken. A resolution was passed, for example, condemning the practice of reducing or remitting the established fees of a college in individual cases. It stated that two consecutive courses of lectures in one year should not entitle students to become candidates for graduation, and resolved that no medical faculty should issue a diploma that did not bear the graduate's name. The new association met annually until 1882, and at each of these meetings, resolutions were passed suggesting ways in which various deficiencies could be corrected. It seems clear that the efforts to raise standards were being pushed too rapidly, for the 1882 meeting in Cincinnati was attended by representatives of only eleven schools. At that time it was deemed best to hold the organization in abeyance.

In 1890, with the pioneering developments in the Johns Hopkins Medical School getting under way, a circular was sent to all American medical colleges announcing another effort to revive the medical school organization and containing an agenda for the meeting. This dealt exclusively with curriculum, and clearly reflects the primitiveness of nineteenth-century medical education. To be discussed were (1) the establishment of a three-year course of six-months each; (2) the need for curriculum to be graded, i.e., basic science before clinical medicine; (3) the institution of written and oral examinations; (4) the establishment of a preliminary examination in the English language; and (5) the need for laboratory instruction in chemistry, histology, and pathology.

This agenda also clearly suggests that the main preoccupation of the AAMC at its inception was curriculum content and management. Areas of concern such as medical care and hospital organization would seem to have been left to the AMA and county medical societies. In any case, virtually all of the colleges that had resigned from the earlier association appeared at this meeting in Nashville. The sixty-six member colleges adopted the new name, "Association of American Medical Colleges." The association began to hold annual meetings in different cities, with the continued emphasis to be focused on the details of students' educational experiences.

Licensing Boards

During the nineteenth century medicine was a pluralistic enterprise. The burgeoning of cults was entirely compatible with the Jacksonian Democracy that characterized the midcentury. Since still-primitive medical science not yet really influenced the ways in which doctors cared for their patients, there seemed little to choose from between these various cults and "regular" medicine. In addition to allopathy, from which sprang modern medicine, these cults included homeopathy, Thomsonian medicine, eclectics, osteopathy, and hydropathy. Quoting Riska, "The question posed by a number of scholars is why sectarian and pluralistic medicine achieved such popularity and strength in the 1830s and 1840s. . . . One major factor was the political and social climate of the Jacksonian era which was characterized by anti-elitist sentiments. In the realm of medicine, this sentiment was expressed as a hostility toward licensing regulations which were seen as a measure to create a privileged elite of regular physicians."[4] Hence, licensing of physicians was discouraged and, indeed, some state legislatures reversed licensing laws during this period.[5]

With the establishment of the AMA in midcentury, "regular" medicine got its act together with the consolidation and improvement of medical education among its major goals. Regulation of medical practice and establishment of licensure as a requirement for practice was part and parcel of this effort. As the industrial revolution took hold after the Civil War, a different public climate also developed and licensing once again seemed appropriate. In 1891 the National Confederation of State Medical Examining Boards, composed of physician members of the AMA, in concord with the previous action of the new AAMC, established a minimum of three years of medical training.[6] The new interest in licensing, a phenomenon of the post-Civil War period, phased comfortably into the impact of the Industrial Revolution, the visits of many physicians to German universities, and the growth of wealth and its availability through the foundations interested in medical care and biomedical science.[7])

The American Medical Association

The American Medical Association, also interested in educational quality in medicine, was becoming active, and, in 1904 established its Council on Medical Education and Hospitals.[8] In a contemporary issue of the *Journal of the American Medical Association* (*JAMA*), some of the basic concerns were discussed by Dr. Arthur Bevan, chair of this council. For example, on page 1470, he stated that "such medical education must be equal to that required in England and Germany." In the section on requirements for admission to medical schools, V. C. Vaughan states, "The schools can set their standards as high as they wish, and beyond and above the schools are the state boards of medical examiners which can act as a second barrier to the admission of the undesirable [sic]" (p. 1471). There continues discussion of proper language requirements— German and Latin were deemed essential. The council soon became active, and in 1906 was seriously planning inspections of various medical schools with a view to identifying those that needed to be closed or otherwise modified. The plan included a qualitative rating of these schools as A, B, or C, with related action to follow.[9] This article describes in detail the condition of various schools, and the action appropriate to take on their behalf.

Thus, at the turn of the century we see a serious collaboration between the AMA, its Council on Medical Education, the AAMC, and the licensing boards to control the quality and quantity of medical education. The quality changes were vital and were epitomized in the standards developing at Johns Hopkins and in reforms in other U.S. universities with medical schools. These changes were stimulated in part by the attitudes and educational sophistication attained by the many physicians in their periods of study in German universities.

This action by the AMA was also instrumental in bringing the major factions of medical practitioners together. The reforms have generally been considered objective and promoting a truly scientific basis for modern medicine and medical education, with high standards. The goal, however, was also to restrict the number of physicians, an item about which both private practitioners and the medical elite could agree although disagreement about intraorganizational policy matters was general. Markowitz and Rosner affirm this position and further add that the two groups united in pushing reform of medical education.

> Each believed that the economic and social situation of individual doctors and the profession in general was discouraging. In part this arose from the general feeling of crisis that permeated the society during the depression of the 1890's. In addition, physicians and other professional groups saw their status and power being eroded and engulfed by the tremendous growth, consolidation, and control of industrial capitalism. Doctors sought to assure their financial security and power through their own organization and reform of medical education.[10]

With higher professional status for physicians linked to reducing their number established as policy, the elitist nature of the effort seems clear. The new wave of medical education, espousing science, more stringent entrance requirements, and increased intellectual performance, while clearly necessary, did meld with the larger political, economic, and social goals of the AMA.

The AAMC, meanwhile, continuing as a member of this coalition to unite regular medicine under the banner of science and education, was meeting regularly and was seemingly becoming involved in more specific attention to details of the schools themselves. During the 1904 annual meeting, at about the same time as the formation of the AMA's Council on Medical Education, a member reported on the current status of medical education, resulting from his visits to nine member colleges. His report was in tabular form, as follows:

Number of schools:
Regular medical schools -------------- 128
Homeopathic medical schools -------- 19
Eclectic medical schools --------------- 10
Physiomedical schools ------------------- 3
Nondescript medical schools ----------- 1
Total 161

Length of medical course:
4 years of 6 months each ------ 6 schools
4 years of 7 months each ---- 19 schools
4 years of 7 $1/2$ months each -- 2 schools
4 years of 8 months each ---- 23 schools
4 years of 8 $1/2$ months each --- 1 school
4 years of 9 months each ---- 15 schools

Total 66

Entrance requirements:
Those of the AAMC ----------- 41 schools
High school diploma ----------- 8 schools
Those of their state board of
medical registration -------- 9 schools

Medical college fees varied from $35 to $200 a year.[11]

It is clear, then, that by the first decade of the twentieth century, most of the schools with membership in the AAMC were reporting some form of four-year educational program, and that regular medicine was on the way to its dominant status. The proprietary schools were still in evidence, however. In his 1908 presidential address, Henry B. Ward stated: "All the evidence at hand indicates a surplus of medical schools in our country, and all agencies join in demanding the elimination of the unfit. No action will add greater strength to the forward movement in medical education than weeding out such as cannot justify their existence."[12]

The Johns Hopkins University was founded in 1876 on the model of the German universities, with research and scholarly achievement destined to characterize the entire institution. Led by President Daniel C. Gilman, the proposed medical school, which was opened in 1895, would be an integral part of the university, with similar goals. In fact, Gilman personally recruited William Welch, an eminent research pathologist recently returned from Germany, as its first department chairman.[13] Indeed, it seems that much of the medical school teaching program had already been roughly planned prior to Welch's arrival. In any case, by the turn of the century the Hopkins model was well on its way to becoming the template for medical education in the United States.

The adoption by the major universities in the United States of the German structure of universities as havens for research as well as education included the entire spectrum of institutional organization and goals. The progression into graduate education with its emphasis on research productivity as a major factor in faculty hiring and promotion became a phenomenon of all of higher education. The adoption of such policies by medical schools would seem to have been a result of association with their parent universities. In response to this academic leadership, the AAMC, whose membership consisted of medical school faculty and administrators, became a guardian of the idea of the central nature of biomedical research, and assisted in structuring pedagogy within the medical schools around research as a central force. There appears to have been agreement in this regard between the leading universities, the AMA, the licensing boards, top medical schools, and the AAMC.

THE PROGRESSIVE ERA (1895 TO 1918)

All of these fast-moving events took place during the historical period known as the Progressive Era. Some knowledge of this period and the intensity of feelings which then characterized much of American society is necessary to an understanding of these developments. The period could be interpreted as the time during which the country was adjusting to the advent of the Industrial Revolution. Great technical advances such as the development of the oil industry, railroads, automobiles, and countless other manifestations of industrial progress led to the acquisition of great wealth and power by a few, and a newly discovered standard of personal income and living by a large segment of the upper and middle classes.

The need for huge numbers of unskilled laborers was met largely through the immigration of Europeans and Asians who settled in industrial cities in quest of the liberty and other attributes of the New World. Minimal wages, however, led to massive poverty and the creation of slums of unprecedented magnitude with accompanying increases in crime, disease, and related social pathology.

This prevalence of disease and other pestilence led to the assumption that many of these medical problems were directly related to the basic social conditions of this population. The creation of health departments—usually under the aegis of local governments largely concerned with such issues as sanitation, environmental conditions, and immunizations to control infectious disease—was an official recognition of this aspect of disease causation. Crowding, poverty, and malnutrition were the variables crying for control, without which important new scientific discoveries could be but poorly applied. Social legislation at local and federal levels, such as bills limiting the employment of children and controlling the length of a day's work, became common. Upper- and middle-class women took interest, and settlement houses in the interest of the poor became popular enterprises.

This period saw the beginnings of the labor movement, with progressive intensity in labor-management relations. Confrontations often became violent, and fatalities during these disturbances were not uncommon. Particularly noteworthy were such events as the Colorado "Ludlow Massacre," which may have been the bloodiest of such battles. With a strike that had begun in 1904, the final confrontation did not occur until 1914, after the deaths of a number of miners and a final accommodation with mine owner John D. Rockefeller.[14]

Meanwhile, the Russian Revolution, with its apparent early success in galvanizing radicals the world-over to often wild celebration, had begun. Emma Goldman was carried to "ecstatic heights." "The radical East Side," she wrote, "lived in a delirium, spending almost all of its time at monster meetings and discussing these matters in cafes, forgetting political differences and brought into close comradeship by glorious events happening in the fatherland."[15] Strong feelings and violence were rife, as antagonism between labor, their unionization movement, and the industrial establishment intensified.

The polarization of society during this period was considerable, with industrialists such as Carnegie, Rockefeller, and Harkness labeled "robber barons" by much of the press and public. Identification of the big foundations as instruments of these corporations was apparent. Major universities, which were steadily supplicating these corporations or their related foundations for funds for their science departments and medical schools, became identified with industry and the wealth accessible therefrom. Since industrial wealth was the most likely source of funding for educational programs based on experimental science, the private universities and medical schools had scarcely any recourse other than to obtain a share of these newly available resources to achieve their stated goals.

The Foundations

As wealth continued to accrue to the leaders of industry, some of them established charitable foundations to provide a means for distributing some of this wealth through the development of policies and programs judged to be socially useful. (One foundation official once told me that these foundations were conceived to assuage corporate feelings of guilt.) Decision making vis-à-vis such grants also tended to include factors which might benefit themselves as well as improve their public image. In any case, a group of foundations became the major extramural source of support for basic research and assured the very survival of many medical schools, especially those in the private sector. Among the more influential of these was the Rockefeller Foundation. Through its newly created branch, the General Education Board, an organizational decision was made in 1902 to provide major support to the new medicine through research and education. A year earlier, the foundation had created the Rockefeller Institute for Medical Research.[16] The role of these foundations has been described in many places, and need not be further developed here. Surely their impact in such projects as development of new schools, establishment of the concept of true full time at Hopkins, and their espousal of the principle of research as a major purpose of the new and reformed medical education are well known. However, the "enthronement"[17] of research may well have been considerably aided and nurtured by one or more of these organizations. Frederick Gates, who became president of the General Education Board, espoused the scientism of the age, and seemed fond of such statements as:

> Do not smile if I often think of the Institute as a sort of theological seminary. But if there is over us all the Sum of All, and that Sum conscious—a conscious intelligent Being, and if that Being has any favorites on this little planet, I must believe that these favorites are made up of that ever enlarging group of men and women who are most intimately and in very truth studying Him and his Ways with men.
>
> In these sacred rooms He is whispering His secrets. . . .
>
> As medical research goes on, therefore, it will find out and promulgate, as an unforeseen by-product of its work, new moral laws and new social laws—new definitions of what is right and wrong in our relations with each other.[18]

Apparently, Gates saw biomedical research as an activity with superhuman—if not mystical—characteristics, one which could ultimately resolve human and interactive problems as well as those that reflected themselves in physical terms. He regarded research as an activity in which success should be awarded ultimate acclaim. It would seem quite possible that he had been indoctrinated into this strong position by some of his acquaintances in medical schools. In the early 1900s the sanctity of research as the premium academic value was already receiving strong support from those sources of funding which enabled the very existence of some reformed medical schools.

In the period between the turn of the century and the end of World War II, numerous foundations such as Carnegie, Grant, Commonwealth, and Kellogg, in addition to the Rockefeller, encompassed nearly the entire source of extramural funding for research and other medical school needs. The majority of innovations—beginning with the Johns Hopkins model and culminating in the post-World War II curriculum revision at Western Reserve, funded by the Commonwealth Fund[19]—were financed and, indeed, partly planned by these institutions. While such initiatives were largely within the great private universities, less ambitious projects were sometimes developed by state medical schools, where it was traditionally difficult to convince legislatures of the need for other than the basic ingredients of educational programs. After my recruitment to start the new College of Human Medicine at Michigan State University, President John Hannah stated the inappropriateness for public universities to make extensive use of the foundations. These income sources were designed expressly to provide basic support for private institutions, which did not generally have the guaranteed income inherent in legislative financial commitments.

Thus, from 1910 through the 1930s, most extramural funding benefited the large private universities and their medical schools, increasing their dependence on the profits of big business for meeting their goals. Boards of trustees were generally drawn from the same pool of industrialists, bankers, and other members of the Eastern industrial establishment, from which were also drawn foundation trustees and officers. The elitism to which the AMA had aspired, therefore, was also extended to the private medical schools through their inextricable link to the foundations and the social milieu of corporate America.

A Word about Physicians and Hospitals

Part and parcel of this total reprofessionalization of physicians was the dramatic elevation of their status within hospitals. These institutions, developing from a nineteenth-century tradition of charity, changed rapidly during the Progressive Era. During the late nineteenth century they had been almost totally controlled by lay trustees who admitted patients and selected physicians to manage them once admitted. Approximately 4,500 hospitals were founded after the Civil War, many under religious leadership. Large, public-supported institutions such as Bellevue, Kings County, New York Hospital, and Massachusetts General Hospital also existed, so that cities such as New York and Boston had the beginnings of good systems. Physicians, however, not permitted to admit their own patients to these hospitals, were not happy with the situation, and massive processes of medical staff reorganization were set in motion. These have been well described by Rosner, Starr, and others,[20] and there seems little reason for extensive development here. Suffice it to say that by 1917 hospitals had become reorganized, often at an increased distance from the poor, with medical staff, rather than trustees, in charge of the admission and care of patients. Hospitals became workshops for physicians and their patients, either under professional control of organized medical staffs in community hospitals, or under the professional control of medical faculty in university hospitals. This development was a major step for physicians in their acquisition of power within the emerging health care system.

Relationships with Public Health

By the beginning of World War I medical practice was firmly established within the private sector. A self-respecting physician lived and succeeded as an independent entrepreneur, with his therapeutic and diagnostic armamentarium increasingly derived from his academic interactions, both during and after his medical school days, and from perusal of an increasingly pervasive and eclectic selection of academically-dominated medical journals. The pragmatics of the past were gradually replaced by translation of university- and industry-based research into useful and effective techniques, medications, and procedures. The emphasis of practice was on the individual patient, with fees established according to the physician's estimate of the value of services delivered, and of the patient's ability to pay.

On the other hand, while also profiting from relevant research findings, the public health establishment's mission was generally concentrated on ministering to the health needs of the underserved poor. While health of the individual patient was part of a health department's concern, its major emphasis was on the health of the larger community. Pollution of air, water, and food were of primary concern and, indeed, such environmental parameters were the only variables capable of modification. It must have seemed that in spite of the recent discovery of the tubercle bacillus, poverty and over-crowding were more relevant contributors to widespread infection by this organism than were findings from the research laboratory. Public health physicians were usually salaried and the services rendered in public health clinics were, and still are, often considered unfairly competitive by the individual private practitioner and by his local medical society. The entire payroll of a health department, including nurses, social workers, and laboratory technicians, was usually a function of local, state, or federal governments. The disaffection with which private physicians and their medical societies regarded the public health establishment was often extreme. This mutual antagonism continues to this day.

The methodology and philosophy of the public health movement was also suspect at the academic level, but probably for different reasons. The reformed medical schools considered research rather than the delivery of health care to the disadvantaged to be the gold standard for medical excellence. Better care and health for all the people would result in due season as research advances were translated into more effective therapeutic agents and better relevant technology. Patient care, then, was clearly given a secondary priority in both student learning and as a criterion for faculty hiring and promotion. Public health—with the welfare of people its highest priority—seemed anti-intellectual in contrast, deserving but scant attention as the new and reformed medical schools established their priorities and organized their faculties. While the Rockefeller Foundation funded the first academic School of Public Health at Hopkins in 1916, it required separateness from the medical school for success. Thus, public health and preventive medicine have been poorly represented on medical faculties to this day. Indeed, in universities in which medical schools and schools of public health exist side-by-side, there is frequently little effective communication between them. This is a partial explanation for the continued difficulty for medical faculties to generate programs or curricula with patient-care or general health issues high on their list of educational priorities.

Town-Gown Relationships

In the development of their academic standards and research orientation, Hopkins and the other university-oriented medical schools were strongly supported by those 15,000 or so physicians returning from periods of study in Germany.[21] In Germany, however, they also discovered physicians enjoying higher standards of living and better social status than that to which they had been accustomed. This presumably also strengthened their preference for private practice over fulltime salaried positions. However, some of these physicians had enjoyed financially favored positions and returned as protagonists of the fulltime academic arrangement. With independent sources of income, they were in better positions to accept the lower fulltime salaries of academe where perquisites such as tenure and guaranteed vacations were an important attraction. Later, the financial inequities between town- and gown-physicians became an enduring problem for both medical school administration and the various branches of the AMA.

Indeed, during the entire interval between the two world wars, the ability to accept the lower income inherent in a career of clinical investigation and medical school teaching was essentially limited to those with outside incomes. There was little extramural support for most research, and what there was came sporadically from foundations, industry, or private donors. My own beginnings in academic medicine were at the end of this period, and clinical research laboratories were characteristically in minimally equipped, obscure nooks of the university-affiliated hospital. In that immediate post-World War II period before the advent of NIH-generated academic financial supports, the inadequate nature of stable university salaries for young clinicians with academic aspirations was such as to discourage that career choice for all but those with outside sources of personal income. Supplementation through part-time private practice was essential, with resulting serious conflict with research and teaching which were the real reasons for choosing an academic career. It was generally understood among my contemporaries that productive academic life tended to be reserved as a viable career for those with independent financial means. For me, after overseas army service, just out of pediatric residency, in the middle of my own antibiotic research project, and married with a small child and living hand-to-mouth, academically incompatible compromises such as a small evening primary care practice and a consultantship at the Philadelphia Naval Hospital were needed to make ends meet. While I was fortunate in forging my own particular academic-administrative life, the likelihood of academic success in the field of infectious disease was essentially foreclosed. A few years later, after the coming of the NIH research training grants program, I would undoubtedly have pursued that academic subspecialty, whether for better or worse. (The history of the growth and development of the NIH will be considered in chapter 3.)

The Flexner Report (1910)[22]

While this document has come to be revered as the turning point through which science and high academic standards were introduced into medical education—and reached almost biblical status for those who were to follow in Abraham Flexner's footsteps—it is clear that much of the evolutionary process had already transpired by the time this report was published. It serves, however, as a beautifully written and incisive statement, both of the inadequacy of proprietary and poorly funded schools and of the inherent excellence of university medical education based largely on the Hopkins model. The work that led to the report was undertaken after the AMA had completed its study of medical schools, and had determined which schools needed to be closed, improved, or maintained.[23] Anxiety, lest the survey be interpreted by the public as self-serving, led to the idea that a similar study by an outside agency might be better received. There was much discussion between Bevan, chair of the AMA Council on Medical Education, and Pritchett, president of the Carnegie Foundation. Some accounts of this relationship credit those discussions with reaching an agreement that a repetition of the AMA inquiry by a foundation would remove any suggestion that the AMA had acted in its own self-interest and confirm that the schools were indeed as they had stated. In any case, the Carnegie Foundation was recruited to do the new study, Dr. Flexner was chosen, and the survey study was done.[24]

The document, as it describes in detail the often miserable conditions under which students struggled in many of these medical schools, fits in well with the popular muck-raking style of the period. More than this, however, it was a discourse on medical education by a highly respected practitioner of innovative education in his own boys' school in Louisville, Kentucky.[25] Flexner's program there had been characterized by an emphasis on the basics such as Greek and Latin, individual attention, and the progress of each student at his own rate. Prior to taking on the medical school study, his own most important reading had been Billroth's "The Medical Sciences in the German Universities." As a graduate of Johns Hopkins, the application of Flexner's own educational expertise to that of medicine was apparently derived mostly from intensive interaction with members of the Hopkins medical faculty, which at that time was also educationally innovative. The model described in the report is essentially that of the Hopkins educational program.

29

The document has often been quoted and misrepresented as one that demanded conformity in medical education, and rigidly emphasized the laboratory sciences during the first two years of medical education. A careful reading of Flexner's writings, however, has shown that in truth such was the intent of neither the author nor the foundation. For example, Flexner states in relationship to the basic sciences,

> ... he needs a different apperceptive and appreciative apparatus to deal with other, more subtle elements ... one must rely for the requisite insight and sympathy on a varied and enlarging cultural experience ... scientific progress has greatly modified his ethical responsibility. His relation was formerly to his patient—and it was almost altogether remedial. But the physician's function is fast becoming social and preventive, rather than individual and curative.[26]
> Later, we read this, concerning lock-step teaching.
> A uniform apportionment between various subjects in schools of the highest grade is neither feasible or desirable. The endeavor to improve medical education through iron clad prescription of curriculum or hours is a wholly mistaken effort.... The prescribed curriculum is a staff upon which those lean who have not strength to walk alone.... Physiology revises and mends anatomy, and the clinical years may be safely relied on to build out here and there the details of pathology.[27]

Such ideas are even more apparent in some of Flexner's later work.[28] It is evident that this distinguished educator, with his basic concepts specifically tailored to medicine, long anticipated the educational research that only recently has begun to be taken seriously by some medical faculties.

Thus, although the Flexner Report and later writings reveal that his message to medical educators was in truth an appeal for flexibility and an exhortation to consider medical education to be preparation for a scientific—yet humanistic—calling, it has persistently been interpreted as the authority for the maintenance of rigidity as the main theme of the "Flexnerian curriculum." The post-Flexnerian era has been characterized by strict adherence to the curriculum in the report, with the basic biological sciences occupying nearly the entire two years of the preclinical program. Indeed, Flexner did oppose the notion of clinical experiences during these two years as irrelevant to the fundamental task of mastering basic science material which, in his view, was the predominant educational substance of the preclinical years. The "learning-by-doing" aspect of the profuse laboratory experience which featured the new emphasis on scientific learning should be sufficiently stimulating for serious medical students. However, he felt that learning should include much of what has come to be known as "philosophy of science," rather than rote memorization of facts. The basic scientists in the Johns Hopkins faculty were apparently fully in accord with these ideas, and placed considerable responsibility on students to learn for themselves. Over time, however, most basic science departments slipped into rote-memorizing-of-facts-through-lectures and a cookbook style of conducting laboratory exercises. By the 1920s Flexner was concerned about these developments, feeling that this was not the kind of scientific education he had proposed, and that rote-memory-based examinations were entirely misplaced in modern medical education.[29]

Nonetheless, the "Flexnerian" curriculum seemed to work well after World War I. I attended Cornell University Medical College from 1937 until 1941, having graduated from Haverford College as a chemistry major. The new molecular-DNA oriented biochemistry had not yet been espoused by the Cornell Department of Biochemistry and the subject, largely a rehash of college physical and organic chemistry, was not difficult for any of us in that class. Physiology was pleasant, and the laboratory relaxed and good fun. The only really difficult subject was anatomy, with many hours of tedious but interesting dissection and, of course, much memorization. It was all manageable, however, and we were quite aware that there would be no significant clinical medicine until the third year. This was a medical school which prided itself on treating students as persons, and the clinical years were a delight, with excellent patient-oriented teaching. Research was always in evidence as an exciting feature, and was presented as needed to enhance understanding of basic and clinical sciences. Curriculum change, to our knowledge, was never an issue. We were quite content with the way we were taught and learned.

It was after World War II, with the explosion in research funding, that the problems developed. The amount of new information, which under the traditional curriculum had to be learned by students, became overwhelming, and the first two years became nightmarish for faculty as well as students. (This issue is discussed in chapters 3 and 4.)

THE AAMC, 1918 THROUGH 1964

The interval from 1918 through 1964, though essentially free of major organizational developments, did see some interesting events. For example, from 1911 through 1922 the AAMC Annual Meeting was always held in Chicago in synchrony with the meeting of the Council on Medical Education and Hospitals of the AMA. In 1912 the AAMC established its Executive Council in place of the previous Judicial Council. At the 1922 meeting it was reported that the cost of medical education ranged from $786 to $1,027, with the average tuition being $187.

In 1925 the AAMC appointed a Commission on Medical Education, directed by Willard Rapplye. In its final report in 1932 the commission stated, for example:

There is a distinct shift in many medical schools now toward placing greater responsibility on the student for his own training in an effort to emphasize learning by the student in contrast to teaching by the faculty.... The new methods are illustrated by the discontinuance of the rigid class system and uniform time and course schedules; the use of small teaching sections; personal contacts between students and instructors; provisions for reasonable free time for reading, individual work, and leisure; a reduction in the amount of lecturing; and opportunities for those who desire, and are competent to do, independent work. These changes are in recognition of the fact that the crucial element is the individual student, upon whose character, attitude, preparation, ability, and industry so largely depend the results of medical training.[30]

Had this report been heeded, it would have greatly benefited medical education. These recommendations more accurately reflected Flexner's advice than did the rigid curricula then the rule and anticipated the outcomes of future studies. That such a report was sponsored by the AAMC, even though not followed by notable innovative activity in the member schools, indicates that there were those who were ahead of their times, and that the AAMC was cautiously attempting to provide constructive leadership.

Indeed, the organization was growing and becoming better equipped to serve its constituent members. The name of the *AAMC Bulletin*, which had started publication as a quarterly in 1926, was changed to the *Journal of the Association of American Medical Colleges* in 1928, and became a bimonthly in 1929. It became the *Journal of Medical Education* in 1950 and in 1989 its name was again changed to *Academic Medicine*. Work was begun on the Medical Colleges Aptitude Test, which was first offered on a single day throughout the nation in 1931; it became a generally required admissions hurdle in 1947. A number of tests, bulletins, and other publications of educational interest appeared, such as the first Applicant Study, based on matriculation questionnaires of all American medical students, and the first Student Accomplishment Records were sent to the 200 colleges that sent students into medicine in 1929. The home office was in Chicago, and the secretary was provided with filing space and adequate assistance in 1932.

During this period, while the association itself was generally supporting the traditional educational approach, speeches given at the annual meetings tended to try to move the organization into different levels of involvement. For example, such topics as "The Danger of the Stereotyped Curriculum" (1923), and "Experiences with Medical Clinics to the First Year Classes" (1924) were presented, and in 1925 all delegates to the annual meeting had an opportunity to visit classes in session at Harvard, Boston University, and Tufts. Two papers dealing with "Correlation between Laboratory and Clinical Teaching" were given at the 1928 meeting, and "A Survey of Several Educational Experiments in American

University Medical Colleges" was heard at the 1930 meeting in Denver.

The Liaison Committee on Medical Education, with three members each from the AAMC and the AMA's Council on Medical Education and Hospitals, was formed in 1942, and the current arrangement for medical school accreditation was under way. The establishment of this committee appears to have engendered some controversy, since the role of accreditor of medical schools was now shared by practitioners with equal votes. It was expected that the committee would meet periodically, that it would develop standards for accreditation, and that its decisions would be final.

In 1953 a category of Individual Memberships in the Association was established; a series of AAMC teaching institutes was begun, and the *Journal* became a monthly publication. In 1955 the association was incorporated, and plans were approved for the building of a central office in Evanston, Illinois. The first longitudinal study of an entire entering class was published in November 1955.

The membership of the association numbered about 1600 in 1956. There were 82 institutional members, 12 affiliates from Canada and the Philippines, 1500 individual, and 7 sustaining members.

The organization's budget included $29,000 for the executive director's office, $67,000 for secretarial and clerical help, $82,000 for journal and publications, $36,000 for a medical audio visual institute, and $154,000 for a committee on educational research and services. Nearly half of the total 1956 budget of $370,000 was committed to educational development and services!

The period between the Flexner Report and the AAMC's move to Evanston with the installation of Ward Darley as its executive director, had generally been one of measured progress during which significant change in medical education or the structure of the AAMC was rarely contemplated. Now, however, things were changing rapidly. A public outcry for an increase in numbers of physicians, the entering of the federal government into medical educational funding, public restiveness with the increasing costs of medical care and the apparent over-specialization of the profession, and the high probability of enormously increased availability of funds from the NIH were among the developments suggesting that a small "deans club" was no longer adequate. In order to facilitate effective responses to the new situation and to foster support of the projected increase in size, numbers, and complexity of medical schools, major reorganization was clearly needed. Action came in 1963 with the appointment of a committee to review the situation and to make recommendations for the appropriate response of the AAMC. The report of this committee, chaired by Lowell Coggeshall, president of the University of Washington, is most readable, with both its style and content giving one the feeling that Flexner himself might have been one of the participants.

THE COGGESHALL REPORT (1965)

The committee serving with Coggeshall consisted of Michael De Bakey, William Hubbard, John Deitrick, Clark Kerr, George Perera, and Robert Berson, then president of the AAMC.[31] The report began with an abbreviated history of the AAMC, medical care, and the accomplishments of the AAMC and the AMA since the 1900s. The current status of medical education was reviewed in its preamble. Since World War II the number of medical graduates had increased from about 6,000 per year to 7,336 in 1964. However, the numbers of housestaff were such that the *New York Times* is quoted as claiming that 60 percent of those in New York were graduates of foreign medical schools. At the end of World War II there were seventy-seven approved schools, with ten new four-year schools established and approved during the postwar period. At the time of the report, in addition, eight four-year schools and three two-year schools were in various stages of planning. However, projections of population increases were such that there seemed no way for the numbers of medical students, even with the planned increases, to be adequate. The report stated that the increase would be achieved both by expansion of existing schools and the development of new institutions, but that the expansion should occur within universities as part of these larger institutions rather than as independent entities.

In order to support this significantly expanded notion of the mission and scope of medical education, implications for the structure and function of the AAMC were significant. These included the need for the association to direct its efforts toward the entire university. This was made essential by the growing interdependence of all aspects of education for health care and medical sciences, other disciplines, and the full scope of physician education.

The report emphasized the mutual needs of both the university and the AAMC. The association could no longer relate itself to deans of medical schools alone and serve medical education effectively. The association should encourage member medical schools to involve themselves more completely and specifically in the affairs of their sponsoring universities. Conversely, the association should provide opportunities for university officials outside the medical school to participate meaningfully in the work of the association.

The report declared the AAMC to be the organization that could most effectively provide needed leadership and serve as spokesman for education for the entire range of health professions and medical sciences. The AAMC, then, would fill the leadership vacuum in this area of professional and educational coordination.

There was considerable elaboration of the services that the AAMC would provide, such as studying basic educational processes and reviewing instruction in the organization and methods dealing with the provision of medical care. There was much emphasis on teamwork in patient care, with the AAMC being the most appropriate organization to represent the coordination needed for effective education for such interdisciplinary behavior.

Financial support of health profession education would be a major task, and an effective and permanent relationship with government would be essential. The federal government would be the main focus of the national organization's attention, and locating where this would be most likely to succeed was one of the considerations of the committee.

In order to facilitate conversion from an organization which had always been dominated by deans to one which included not only the entire spectrum of medical education but also their parent universities, recommendations for extensive organizational modification were developed.[32] The following is a brief summary of these recommended changes.

First, a name change was proposed to reflect more accurately the subsidiary nature of medical education within the greater university and its championship of interdisciplinary teaching. Something like "Association for the Advancement of Medical Education" was suggested. Institutional membership would extend beyond the medical school, and be defined as "institutions maintaining medical colleges." Within the organization, the following summarizes relevant structural recommendations.

The General Assembly would be composed of three representatives selected by each institution: the university's chief executive officer, the medical school dean, and a member of the medical faculty with broad interest in education for health and medical sciences. There would also be membership from such affiliate and related organizations as the AMA and the American Nursing Association.

The General Assembly would be the site of governance of the association, and would perform such tasks as elect the Executive Council, adopt and amend by-laws, establish standards for accreditation, and approve major programs. Thus, the AAMC would become democratically governed. The officers would include a chairman elected annually by the General Assembly and, for the first time in the AAMC's history, a full-time president.

The Executive Council, also elected by the General Assembly but heavily weighted toward medical school deans, would also include two representatives of other institutional members, one of whom should be a general university officer.

There would be three Advisory Councils: the **Council of Deans**, primarily concerned with educational matters and with internal administration of medical colleges, would also be concerned with relationships of the medical colleges to other elements of the university. The **Council of Administrators** would consist of all member university presidents, or their representatives, and would be con-

cerned with the administration and financing of physician education and with health and medical sciences as a part of the total
university. The **Council of Faculty** would provide for participation
of faculty representatives selected for their broad interest in education for health and medical sciences. This council should be concerned primarily with matters of curriculum, educational content,
and teaching methods.

These three councils would be very influential in the governance
of the organization; again, though, the subsidiary relationship of
the medical dean to the university president is made clear.

There would be three commissions at a lower level than the councils which would provide opportunities for direct participation of
affiliate members in matters of particular interest to them and related organizations. They should not have legislative prerogatives.
These would be **Related Health Organizations, Teaching Hospitals**, and **Teaching Organizations**. For our purposes the most important of these was the recommendation for the Teaching Hospitals, which apparently were deliberately not accorded the status of
deans or faculty of medical schools.

In addition, some form of regionalization was recommended to
provide more access to institutions as well as more frequent deliberations relevant to local situations. The recommendation was also
made that, in order to be more effective with the federal establishment, the Association should establish its headquarters in Washington, D.C.

The report reads as though it were a direct expression of the
substance of the Flexner's *Bulletin Number Four*. However, the
document was accepted by the AAMC as its blueprint for the future
only after a harrowing and often bitter debate, and after the following changes were imposed.

1. The name change was rejected, and the Association of American Medical Colleges would continue.
2. Institutional memberships remained the medical schools.
3. The Council of Administrators was abandoned.
4. The Council of Faculty became the Council of Academic Societies, perpetuating disciplinary and departmental status for
   faculty at the national level. A number of disciplines other
   than those recommended by the committee were added.
5. The teaching hospitals were elevated to council level.
6. The other commissions (related health organizations and
   teaching organizations) were eliminated.
7. The Organization of Student Representatives (OSR) was established.

Thus, the Coggeshall Report was approved and adopted by the
AAMC only after the association's deliberative process reduced
many of its recommendations to its own self-image. Indeed, while

the report's suggestions for expansion were enthusiastically endorsed, the main specific suggestion accepted was the move to Washington, D.C. which, as was intended, did improve the association's access to the federal government. Otherwise, however, the retention of institutional memberships within the medical schools may have catalyzed further separation from the universities themselves. The denial of council status to university presidents excluded them from significant participation in national concerns of medical education, and the establishment of the Council of Academic Societies (CAS) facilitated an ever-increasing preoccupation with research and specific funding and organizational concerns of their individual disciplines. Generally, it became a bastion of the traditional modes of teaching and student evaluation rather than the education-oriented group intended by the original report.

The establishment of the Council of Teaching Hospitals (COTH) in lieu of the committee's recommendation of the lower status of "commission" was also an important step in the development of the next chapter in the history of American medical education. The decades ahead would be ones in which the provision of medical care and the mechanisms for its funding would become of increasing significance to medical colleges, most of which either controlled or owned their teaching hospitals. Having equal status with medical college deans and faculties in the AAMC organization would seem to have enabled hospital administrators to influence AAMC policy more effectively. Leaders in the teaching hospital world would become members of the Executive Council and chairmen of the General Assembly. Much of the AAMC's dealings with Congress would have to do with such issues as Medicare payments for hospitalization and for reimbursement of clinical faculty. The entire concept of a medical school, indeed, would metamorphose into the idea of the "Academic Medical Center," whose very name stresses the functional diversity of these increasingly huge medical complexes. Of necessity, issues of education became sublimated to the needs of the entire medical center, and in some of these institutions medical student education could almost be considered a byproduct of the entire system. This is not to imply that education disappeared from she agendas of medical schools or the AAMC: it simply means that the responsibilities of deans, faculties, and hospital administrators became increasingly diffuse, and were appropriately reflected in the organizational pattern and preoccupations of the AAMC staff and academic leadership.

The advent of the OSR has had a considerable impact, since the students selected to membership participate actively in annual meetings, and their contribution is formalized in discussions in the General Assembly as well as in meetings of the councils.

Subsequently, the AAMC moved to comfortable quarters in Washington, D.C., its first fulltime president was elected and installed, and effective staff development began. The annual meetings became huge and were increasingly characterized by meetings of subgroups such as student affairs, business managers, and Research in Medical Education. Plenary sessions became uniformly formal, interesting, and topical, featuring public and political figures as well as leaders in medical education. The event, alternating annually between Washington, D.C. and other major cities, is useful as a site for faculty recruitment, formal or informal meetings, and as host to related academic organizations such as the Society for Health and Human Values, and the Association for Hospital Medical Education. The annual meeting is fun, informative, and serves both formally and informally as an important meeting place for all levels of those involved in American medical education.

Since the qualified acceptance of the Coggeshall Report, the AAMC has emerged as a large and powerful organization with enormous influence over the nature of the academic medical center, the structure of curriculum and, inevitably, over the quality and style of American medical care. The political stance of its policies, its attitudes about academic values and evaluation, and its positions on goals of student progress and career outcomes are all intensely significant in shaping programmatic structure and ambience in its member institutions.

We have described how broad and visionary proclamations from the dais at annual meetings, AAMC Institute conclusions, and study reports usually failed to influence traditional educational policy in the pre-Coggeshall period. We have also seen how some significant liberalizing features of the Coggeshall Committee's blueprint for AAMC expansion and development were rejected during the debate leading to its "acceptance" by the membership. Activities either impinging on the AAMC or actually initiated by the organization have continued to test its flexibility during the past two decades. Two such important events were the GAP and the GPEP reports.

EVALUATION IN THE CONTINUUM OF MEDICAL EDUCATION: REPORT OF THE COMMITTEE ON GOALS AND PRIORITIES OF THE NATIONAL BOARD OF MEDICAL EXAMINERS—THE "GAP" REPORT[33]

Evaluation of student progress is a matter of intense and often emotional disagreement throughout the field of education. Medical education has been no exception, and an in-depth discussion of this subject is not the purpose of this book. Nor will technical issues such as multiple-choice versus essay examination structure be discussed. The importance of the issue lies in the oft-repeated statement that "as students are examined, so will they learn."[34] Hence, examination policy which assumes rote memorization of facts for successful performance will promote that sort of learning. On the other hand, examinations concentrating on problem solving and basic principles reinforce learning programs which cultivate such analytical thinking. It is the latter approach which seems to have characterized the basic science faculty in the early years of Hopkins, and which Flexner really favored in his various writings. Over the years, however, teaching and examination policies have leaned toward the mode of rote memorization at both basic science and clinical levels. One effect has been the tendency for medical students to view the learning of basic science during the two preclinical years as a necessary and unpleasant hurdle to be jumped before getting on with the real business of medicine.

State licensing boards have generally constructed their examinations in accord with this style, with their tests divided into separate preclinical and clinical areas. The National Board of Medical Examiners[35] was created in 1915 to develop a national alternative to the multiple, and often confusing, state-dominated licensing tests. The complex interaction between the NBME and the state boards is referred to in the well-referenced works here cited. The NBME staff has retained the traditional dichotomy between basic sciences (Part I) and the clinical subjects (Part II) with subject-specific examination questions contributed by medical school faculty. The state-of-the-art National Board examinations have come to be accepted by most state boards and, with the advantage of nearly total national validity, have become almost uniformly the first choice for licensing purposes of both medical faculties and students.

However, not always to the delight of the National Board staff, their original objective as tests for licensure has been subverted by use in medical schools as instruments to measure the effectiveness of curricula. This tendency has led to pressure from the accrediting agency for medical schools to require these examinations as benchmarks of student progress. Strong and often competitive stress can become part of the second-year student's life as he or she strives to excel in these tests to support the institution's cumulative score. It is often the case that schools require passing Part I of the National Boards at the end of the second year as a gateway to admission to the clinical years. Those who favor such a requirement, generally basic scientists, feel that such well-conceived tests, created by experts in the testing field, are the best available means for ascertaining the effectiveness of their teaching methods and execution. In their view, such rigorous examinations are the best way to be certain that the students have, in fact, learned what they should know in order to enter the clinical years. Abandoning such an exercise, then, would be an anti-intellectual step inappropriate to medical education.

Those who oppose this approach think that it turns the first two years of medical school into a cram course for the National Boards, seriously hampering the introduction of clinical, ethical, and other humanistic subjects that are considered vital in today's world of medical care. Furthermore, with success in Part I requiring mostly rote memorization of facts, the self-learning and problem-solving needs of physicians are not well tested. Far better might be the dropping of Part I, and the substitution of a combined examination upon graduation in which the relationships between basic science and clinical phenomena would be among the major emphases of the testing procedure. This academic group seems to be reiterating the conclusions of Flexner, as he compared unfavorably the American tendency for periodic memory-testing with the European style of comprehensive examinations emphasizing scientific principles more than factual details.

In any case, the NBME questioned the use of their examinations as curriculum evaluating mechanisms, and instituted a study culminating in the publication of the *GAP Report* in 1973. The study committee was chaired by William D. Mayer, M.D., and was composed of thoughtful educators as well as the director of Academic Affairs at the AAMC.

In recognizing the negative impact of NBME examinations on interdepartmental teaching, the resulting study noted that the same level of science may not be needed by all students, and that the basic responsibility of medical school is to prepare students for residency. While intended as a ten-year plan that could lead to the NBME to assume evaluation responsibilities for the entire continuum of medical education, it was widely assumed that the report was a signal for the immediate implementation of its recommendations. The suggestion that caused the most alarm among many deans and medical scientists was that calling for a "Qualifying A" examination at the interface between medical school and residency to certify the students' ability to practice under supervision in the residency setting. The alarm resulted largely from the assumption that this presaged the abolition of Part I of the National Boards, with possible serious anti-intellectual consequences.

The debate on this subject in the Council of Deans was intense. I well remember such a discussion at the council's spring meeting at that time. By and large, the arguments in favor of retaining Part I as a measure both of successful preclinical learning and of curricular validity was upheld by the deans of established research-rich academic medical centers. Those of us from newer institutions, with perhaps more intense interest in educational philosophy, emphasized the negative impact of such a test on student progress in programs stressing a smooth flow of learning throughout the entire four years. Reimposing this test simply would perpetuate the fallacy of separation of basic sciences from clinical medicine, and would dilute efforts to leaven the preclinical years with relevant clinical and humanistic considerations. We had little impact, however, on the debate's resolution. The National Board's notion of a single qualifying examination at the time of the awarding of the M.D. degree was not supported. Part I remains a requirement at the termination of the second year in most medical schools, with student grade levels often a major topic of scrutiny by both accreditation teams and the Liaison Committee itself in its accreditation-related decisions.

PHYSICIANS FOR THE TWENTY-FIRST CENTURY: REPORT OF THE PANEL ON THE GENERAL PROFESSIONAL EDUCATION OF THE PHYSICIAN (1984)[36]

Throughout its history, both in its own proceedings and in its accreditation-related association with the AMA, the AAMC has been heavily involved in matters of academic standards and curriculum form and function in its member medical schools. It has been noted that with the expansion of medical school areas of responsibility—and the AAMC's derivative staffing expansion and need to be increasingly pervasive in its expertise—there appears to have been some understandable dilution of interest in and concern for details of curriculum. However, the AAMC has continued to support the section on Research in Medical Education (RIME) both with appropriate staff and generous allocation of time and space at each annual meeting. Thus, under the aegis of the AAMC much progress, which has not really been recognized by the actions of the LCME in its accreditation decisions, has been made in the field. Perhaps in recognition of this situation, and of the need for the AAMC to be out front so far as educational programming was concerned, the study on the General Professional Education of the Physician was undertaken.

Commissioned as an official activity of the AAMC and funded by the Henry J. Kaiser Family Foundation, this study and its report, published in 1984, was one of the AAMC's most comprehensive undertakings. Hearings were held in various parts of the United States by director Steven Muller, then president of Johns Hopkins University, and comments were solicited from representatives of all U.S. and Canadian medical schools, as well as from colleges and universities, medical professional societies, and other groups.

The report was prepared after the following working groups had completed their deliberations: essential knowledge, fundamental skills and personal qualities, values, and attitudes. Each group met three times and submitted written reports to the Project Panel. These reports were published in the *Journal of Medical Education* (part 2) in November 1984.[37] In addition to the three working groups, reports were made by six subgroups of the working group on fundamental skills in the areas of clinical skills, learning skills, medical information science skills, critical appraisal skills, application of the scientific method, teamwork skills, and personal management skills.

While the comprehensiveness of the approach is unquestioned, it is surprising that medical ethics and jurisprudence were apparently not represented on the panel. Since a huge share of the difficult issues in medical care include medical liability, informed consent, and matters of technological excesses in the care of elderly and fatally ill patients, attention to such problems would seem to have been essential. Otherwise, it is hard to fault the nature of the participants or their conclusions and recommendations.

In brief, the report recommended the adoption of such pedagogical principles as de-emphasizing rote learning, lectures, and high technology medicine in favor of problem solving, self-learning, and clinical concentration on patients and families. It called for each school to develop an identifiable budget for educational programs, and dealt with numerous other subjects with a generally constructive educational view.

Recognizing the critical nature of accreditation in implementing this report, a relevant section states:

> If the AAMC and its Canadian equivalent] were to emphasize that the purposes of general professional education are to select and educate students to be active, independent learners, and to prepare them for specialized graduate medical education, the dominance of memorization and recall in medical education would be reduced and program changes commensurate with the conclusions and recommendations in the report could be accomplished.[38]

This statement could be interpreted as a challenge to the LCME to encourage appropriate implementation of relevant aspects of this report in its accreditation decisions, and as recognition that successful implementation would be unlikely without assistance from the accreditation process.

However, at the 1984 annual meeting, a hearing was held by the LCME on the content of the new accreditation guidelines entitled "Functions and Structure of a Medical School."[39] The question was asked from the floor as to the LCME's intent vis-à-vis GPEP, which had been the main feature of the generally favorable plenary session on the preceding day. The response was to the effect that the LCME would not take leadership in this matter. Rather, it would stay within its guidelines and modify them appropriately should the suggested educational changes really become apparent.

In his "Afterword" to the report, John Cooper, then president of the AAMC, called attention to the 1933 Rapplye Commission Report[40] and noted that its recommendations were not implemented, and that it would be up to the medical schools themselves, rather than the AAMC, to push the new effort.

One year later, at the 1985 annual meeting, a document adopted by the Executive Council entitled "Commentary on the GPEP Report" was circulated.[41] While moderate in tone, nowhere did it express enthusiasm for the report, and it identified the problems for department chairmen and deans. For example:

Within each medical school, some faculty members will be more involved with medical students than others. Faculty members who carry major responsibility for the curricular functions of a school should not be exempt from other scholarly contributions. While sacrificing the quantity or rate of research productivity, they must not sacrifice the quality of their scholarly contributions. These faculty members may encounter difficulty in acquiring support for their research; leaders in institutions and foundations are encouraged to develop mechanisms that will assist them in sustaining research programs having limited rates of productivity.[42]

Here, then, the fear of yielding ground on the side of teaching over research in the continuing struggle between these two basic faculty tasks is clearly expressed. Without maintaining productivity in acceptable academic scholarship (usually defined as bench research) a truly successful academic career is proclaimed to be unlikely.

The commentary worried about the implications of specific budgeting for education, and suggested that deans and department chairmen must provide leadership for the educational function of their schools, and to foster this goal

the COD-CAS Working Group believes it is desirable that the major committee charged with the responsibility for the overall design and coordination of the curriculum should be composed of departmental chairmen. Interdisciplinary committees and individual faculty members, operating in a coordinated fashion, can schedule and implement the curriculum, based on established policies.[43]

This section asserted that faculty with administrative titles should lead the school through the major curriculum changes. Presumably, this would guard against irresponsible faculty decision making, and protect the high status of research.

This official AAMC response to one of its major studies of national attitudes about the quality of education in American medical schools falls back on the administrative dilemma which ensues when education is identified as a primary institutional objective. Under such conditions, money targeted for research may need to be reallocated in favor of education. Talented faculty members must be more involved in teaching at the expense of research productivity, and implications for decreased extramural research funding are apparent. Finally, anxiety about turning this entire emphasis on education over to faculty resulted in the notion that departmental chairpersons should remain in control, assuring that significant alterations in administrative priorities would occur only with great difficulty.

This position, furthermore, appears to contradict what I have always considered to be the appropriate relationship between administration and faculty. Under this philosophy, the dean, probably with the assent of his department chairs, establishes the general educational goals, and describes the administrative constraints and the general context of space and budget possibilities. If there are foreseeable administrative accommodations which might need to be made, these are identified. A charge is then developed for the appropriate ad hoc or permanent faculty committee (whether departmental or collegewide) to develop recommendations for the curriculum alteration which then must be submitted to faculty for approval. Within affected departmental and plenary faculty meetings on the subject, chairs and the deans office can express their administrative ideas of feasibility; the basic academic responsibility, however, resides with faculty. Once accepted as college or departmental policy, it is then within the duties of the administration to effect scheduling, financing, staffing, and other modifications needed to implement the faculty-developed curricular changes.

It will be interesting to follow the impact of this report. That it has been and will continue to stimulate discussion and serve as the base for change in medical schools seems clear. For example, coincidentally with the 1987 AAMC annual meeting, the Generalists in Medical Education met in a nearby hotel in Washington, D.C. with a program featuring the AAMC's vice president for Academic Affairs, and dealing to a large extent with GPEP-type issues.[44] The meeting, usually in well attended small sessions, dealt mainly with programs utilizing innovative teaching methods. But few deans or department chairs were present and it was readily admitted that, without space and budget allocation, the capacity of groups such as these to make a significant impact is seriously limited. Occasional papers in such periodicals as the *Journal of Medical Education* (now *Academic Medicine*) are also suggestive of some movement in this direction.

Indeed, the likelihood of such an event is presently unclear. The new president of the AAMC—who is greatly interested in the apparent surplus of American physicians, is aware of the problems that have clouded the accreditation process, and who wants to make important changes—has been in office for about two years. A controversial director of accreditation resigned and has been replaced. The president's recent speeches are encouraging changes in clinical teaching, and the AAMC is currently engaging in workshops for schools that are considering adopting problem-oriented curricula. An excellent and encouraging recent AAMC publication describes not only the general and specific status of American medical education but also directs attention to the need for change.[45] In the context of answering the question: "Will medical school faculties be able to adopt instructional methods that more actively involve students in the learning process?" it describes the current foundation-supported project, Assessing Change in Medical Education (ACME). This study is designed to determine how change in medical education programs has occurred in response to the GPEP report. In addition, the publication calls attention to the need for high priorities to be assigned to such issues as the underrepresentation of minorities in medicine, medical care of the aging population, and the complexities of the AIDS epidemic. The 1989 one-hundredth anniversary annual meeting likewise reflected the AAMC's seriousness about such change-oriented program. As well as containing the usual financial and anecdotal review of the year's work, the AAMC's *1988–89 Annual Report*,[46] stresses such issues as the need for an increased emphasis on rural health care.

The ambience and general content of the report of the 1989 annual meeting has been refreshing and encouraging. One gets the impression that the AAMC leadership feels the urgency of the need for change. The president's address at the opening plenary session was a powerful plea for dramatic change in both structure and content along the lines of increased student responsibility, essentially abandoning the current notion of the fourth educational year, and a generally increased emphasis on primary care. His final statement cautioned against compromising "quality." Therein, of course, could lie the rub. If quality continues to be defined mostly through such measures as student grades in National Board, Part I examinations, and the degree to which a school succeeds in expanding the scope of high-technology tertiary care in its medical center, little real change can be expected. It seems to me that full endorsement by the AAMC power structure of the president's call to action—as expressed in the Executive Council, the CAS, COD, and COTH—is a necessary condition to effecting real change. Such an endorsement could lead to a redefinition of educational and institutional quality that could encompass the broadened purpose of our medical schools. Favorable decisions by the LCME would signal both necessary and sufficient conditions for substantive medical school change, influential AAMC appointees to this body could then convert it to an agency supporting and monitoring relevant institutional change, as well as guarding the public against victimization by inadequately educated physicians.

A point that will be reiterated later in this monograph is the need for more flexibility in the accreditation process. For example, there would seem to be little reason to force a primary care or rural health program on an established medical school with an excellent tertiary-care-oriented medical center and outcome goals for its graduates focused around careers in traditional academic research-oriented medicine. On the other hand, a semirural institution with a mission statement clearly including rural and small town primary care might well be censured for attempting to duplicate the high-tech expertise of its urban counterpart. The LCME, however, might also pressure such a school to pioneer in the development of scholarly research in the solution of problems incidental to its stated primary goals and to adjust its criteria for appointment and promotion of faculty accordingly.

The difficulties inherent in such a transformation should not be underestimated. Ever since Flexner—and even more so since the post-World War II infusion of research funds, training grants, and increasing opportunities for careers in investigation and academic specialization—the paradigm for academic success has been almost exclusively based on research accomplishment, scientific knowledge, and technical skill. Resentment of "softer" criteria for academic effectiveness is entirely understandable, especially in view of the extraordinarily high esteem with which these traditional values are held not only by academe but by much of the general public. The very life-blood of extramural funding of the modern medical center is that provided by the NIH and by income from high-cost tertiary medical care; there is currently but little to be found for educational development. The solution to such problems will require imaginative leadership at all levels of medical academe and at such levels as political action and reeducation of the public vis-à-vis its relationship to the academic medical center.

The ensuing chapters will deal with more specific discussions of curricular developments, the impact of the huge growth of research funding on medical education, and the accreditation process. The overall theme of the discussion will continue to emphasize the dependence of the quality of health and medical care on leadership from academic medicine, and the quality, attitudes, and behavior of the physicians over whose entire professional lives academe exerts such a huge influence.

NOTES

1. Lowell Coggeshall, *Planning for Medical Progress through Education* (Evanston, Ill.: Association of American Medical Colleges, 1965).
2. Exceedingly readable and well referenced is, of course, Paul Starr's *The Social Transformation of American Medicine* (New York: Basic Books, 1982), 112–13.
3. Dean F. Smiley, "History of the Association of American Medical Colleges," *Journal of Medical Education* 32, no. 7 (1957): 512–25.
4. Elianne Riska, *Power, Politics and Health: Forces Shaping American Medicine* (Helsinki: Finnish Society of Sciences and Letters, 1985).
5. Richard D. Shryock, *Medical Licensing in America, 1650–1965* (Baltimore: The Johns Hopkins University Press, 1967), 55–56.
6. Walter L. Bierring, "Medical Licensure after Forty Years," *Federation Bulletin* 43, no. 4 (1956).
7. Ibid., "Early Licensing and Subsequent Decadence: 1650–1875," chapt. 1, especially 26–31.
8. Arthur D. Bevan, "Council on Medical Education of the American Medical Association," *JAMA* 44, no. 18 (1905): 1470–75.
9. Ibid., "Council on Medical Education of the American Medical Association," *JAMA* 48, no. 20(1907): 1701–7.
10. Susan Reverby and David Rosner, eds., *Health Care in America: Essays in Social History* (Philadelphia: Temple University Press, 1979), chapt. 10.
11. Smiley, 518.
12. Ibid., 519.
13. Donald Fleming, *William H. Welch and the Rise of Modern Medicine* (Baltimore: The Johns Hopkins University Press, 1954).
14. Page Smith, *America Enters the World*, vol. 7 (New York: McGraw-Hill Book Company, 1985), 391–402. This book provides a good background for the period. Also, E. R. Brown, *Rockefeller Medicine Men* (Berkeley: University of California Press, 1979. A critical and interesting book on the era, and on the role of the foundations and others leading to the Flexner Report.
15. Smith, 65.
16. Kenneth M. Ludmerer, *Learning to Heal: The Development of American Medical Education* (New York: Basic Books, Inc., 1985), 105. He refers there to the following book as the standard reference on the Institute: George W. Corner, *A History of the Rockefeller Institute, 1901–1953, Origins and Growth* (New York: Rockefeller Institute Press, 1964).
17. Ludmerer, 217–18.
18. "Memoirs of Frederick T. Gates," *American Heritage* 6, no. 3 (1955): 73–74.
19. For an exhaustive history of the Commonwealth Fund, see A. McGehee Harvey and Susan L. Abrams, *For the Welfare of Mankind: The Commonwealth Fund and American Medicine* (Baltimore: The Johns Hopkins University Press, 1986).
20. David Rosner, *A Once Charitable Enterprise: Hospitals and Health Care in Brooklyn and New York, 1885–1912* (Cambridge: Cambridge University Press, 1982); and Paul Starr.
21. Thomas N. Bonner, *American Doctors and German Universities.: A Chapter in International Intellectual Relations, 1870–1914* (Lincoln: University of Nebraska Press, 1963).

22. Abraham Flexner, *Medical Education in the United States and Canada: A Report to the Carnegie Foundation for the Advancement of Teaching, Bulletin Number Four* (Boston: The Merrymount Press, 1910).

23. "Council on Medical Education of the AMA, the Chairman, Dr. A. D. Bevan, Presiding," *JAMA* 58, no. 20 (1907): 1701–7.

24. Numerous studies on the AMA-Carnegie Foundation relationship have been done. These were well summarized by Robert Hudson, M.D. in a symposium in Chicago, Illinois, June 10–11, 1986, entitled "Flexner and the 1990s." While the resulting publication has yet to appear, his references include such works as: Carleton Chapman, "The Flexner Report by Abraham Flexner" *Daedalus* 103 (1974): 105–17; Howard Berliner, "New Light on the Flexner Report: Notes on the AMA-Carnegie Foundation Background," *Bulletin of History of Medicine* 51 (1977): 603–9; and Daniel Fox, "Recent Marxist Interpretations of the History of Medicine in the United States," *Clio Medica* 16 (1982): 225.

25. Abraham Flexner, *"I Remember." The Autobiography of Abraham Flexner* (New York: Simon and Schuster, 1940).

26. Flexner, *Bulletin No. Four*, 26.

27. Ibid., 76.

28. Abraham Flexner, *Medical Education, A Comparative Study* (New York: MacMillan Company, 1925).

29. Ibid., 278.

30. "Physicians for the Twenty-First Century, The GPEP Report." (Washington, D.C.: Association of American Medical Colleges, 1984), 35. This is part of the summary statement by John A. D. Cooper, then president of the AAMC.

31. Coggeshall.

32. It should be noted that the entire sequence on the three studies supported by the AAMC, including the Coggeshall Report, the GAP Report, and the GPEP Report, are taken, with but minor modifications, from my talk, "The Impact of Abraham Flexner upon Teaching in American Medical Schools" given at a symposium entitled "Flexner and the 1990's" in Chicago, June 10–11, 1986.

33. "Evaluation in the Continuum of Medical Education," Report of the Committee on Goals and Priorities of the National Board of Medical Examiners, Philadelphia, 1973.

34. See, for example, Flexner, *Medical Education, A Comparative Study*, 279–80.

35. See William G. Rothstein, *American Medical Schools and the Practice of Medicine* (New York: Oxford University Press, 1987), p. 149; and Ludmerer, *Learning to Heal*, 241.

36. Flexner, *Medical Education, A Comparative Study*, 279–80.

37. "Physicians for the Twenty-First Century: The GPEP Report," Report of the Panel on the General Professional Education of the Physician and the College Preparation for Medicine (Washington, D.C.: Association of American Medical Colleges, 1984).

38. *Journal of Medical Education*, Part Two (November 1984).

39. The GPEP Report, 28.

40. Liaison Committee on Medical Education, *Functions and Structure of a Medical School. Standards for Accreditation of Medical Education Programs Leading to the M.D. Degree* (1985).

41. Physicians for the Twenty-First Century, "Commentary on the GPEP Report," adopted by the Executive Council of the Association of American Medical Colleges, September 12, 1985.
42. Ibid., 6.
43. Ibid.
44. "Implementing GPEP," the Eighth Annual Conference for Generalists in Medical Education, November 8 and 9, 1987, Embassy Row Hotel, Washington, D.C.
45. Association of American Medical Colleges, "American Medical Education: Institutions, Programs, and Issues," an AAMC staff report prepared by Robert F. Jones, Ph.D., Director of Institutional Studies, Division of Planning and Development, 1989.
46. "Academic Medicine Faces the Future," Association of American Medical Colleges, 1988–89 Annual Report.

3
Medical Schools and Curricular Innovation

The professional issues which physicians must face—pain, anxiety, fear, death, and all the irrationalities characterizing illness—call for exquisitely personal, patient-oriented processing of data and correspondingly thoughtful diagnostic and therapeutic plans, at once scientific and humanistic. Despite the nearly universal political conservatism of American physicians, one might still expect their scientific education and training to provide the necessary objectivity to act as a liberal force in guiding their diagnoses, treatment, and professional attitude. "Liberal" is used here as meaning unbiased consideration of relevant information regardless of the ideological or disciplinary nature of its source.

It must be remembered, however, that the science which motivates modern medicine is imbued with the conviction that the true cause of disease has been or ultimately will be discovered and effectively treated through the results of biomedical research, and is explainable in mechanistic terms. True causation by a presumed etiological agent, or the therapeutic effectiveness of a new drug can be determined only through statistically significant results from carefully designed research, and double-blind clinical investigation. Such rigid criteria may have the effect of denying the validity of psychologically, socially, or environmentally derived concepts of disease causation; such notions of etiology of illness, falling within the intellectual domain of "soft" social sciences or humanities, are accepted by most physicians at best as temporary hypotheses of possible usefulness until the "real" explanation comes along. While this belief system and methodology has sparked the vast majority of modern medical triumphs, and have served to protect the public from quackery and inadequate medical practice, unqualified dedication to such criteria for medical decision making can tend not only to professional rigidity but also to incomplete and inadequate patient care.

While meticulous attention to scientific validity is fundamental

51

to most of the precision and effectiveness of modern medicine, it can put the patient in a position of being less interesting than the mechanism of the disease from which he or she may be suffering. The patient with the more "interesting" disease tends to take precedent over one with less fascinating signs, symptoms, or biochemical abnormalities. While it is true that the Hippocratic oath—or some modern substitute—to which all physicians must theoretically adhere, provides some sort of basis for an ethical doctor-patient relationship, and a good "bedside manner" and being nice to patients is generally expected, acquisition of such behavior is essentially left to chance, with the relevant behavioral and social sciences and humanities awarded minimal status during the educational process. That many physicians do acquire such a propitious amalgam of medical science and humanism is fortunate; however, the majority public opinion seems to perceive decreasing humanism in the doctor-patient relationship.

While the AMA espouses strict adherence to medicine as science, and while a scientific educational background appears compatible with the fierce individuality and political conservatism of the practicing physician, the AMA has been active in the family practice movement, supporting innovative educational programs in such areas as community medicine and student preceptorships in family physicians' offices. It has also been noted that AMA members of the Liaison Committee on Medical Education (LCME) tend to offset the fundamentally scientific position of those who represent the AAMC in the process of accreditation of medical schools. It is also true that there is far from universal acceptance by practicing physicians of the entire package of AMA ideological and organizational precepts. Many practicing physicians, as AMA members, have joined HMOs, hold salaried positions in universities, government, or industry, and are more liberally inclined vis-à-vis public involvement in financing medical care.

In like fashion, some dissident and innovation-oriented medical faculty have become frustrated by educational traditionalism which, many believe, is at the root of a large part of today's trouble between medicine and the American public. Much of the post-World War II progress in medical education has been generated by these educational innovators, sometimes with the assistance of progressive practitioners and in collaboration with other university-based disciplines such as education, psychology, anthropology, sociology, economics, philosophy, and history. After World War II, some medical faculties within universities began to explore progress in general education, and wondered why medical schools were not using some of the new methodology that might well be relevant to medical education. At the beginning of this new educational era, much attention was focused on the preclinical years, where standard medical school teaching methods consisted largely of lectures, memorization, cookbook laboratory exercises, and examinations that generally concentrated on factual recall. While such methods had worked during an earlier period, the information explosion had by now transformed both teaching and learning into an all-but-impossible task. Departments were demanding more hours; if such leeway were not available, lecturers would simply have to talk faster. Faculty and student frustration became virtually universal. The public by now was also beginning to call attention to the decreasing availability of primary care physicians and to express disenchantment with the apparent decline of personal attention in specialized care. In short, the need for change in the way physicians were educated was becoming apparent from many quarters.

Educational research had long been indigenous to schools and colleges of education, where significant advance in the science and practice of teaching and learning was taking place. It became clear that the idea of "teaching" as effective faculty-expended energy to a passive student was a myth, and that students are not "taught." Rather, students "learn," with faculty as a catalyst to the learning process. Among the first publications applying academic educational research principles to medical education was that of George Miller and his collaborators in 1961.[1] Educational research data were showing that if taught in the traditional fashion, subjects like anatomy were soon forgotten, but that retention was more likely if the material were presented in the context of clinical relevance. Faculty interest in theory and practice of modern pedagogy became widespread, and coincided with the public pressure for the system to expand both numbers and qualifications of its graduates. Federal and foundation funds were soon to become available for expansion of existing schools, creation of new ones, and for research in medical education.

EDUCATIONAL INNOVATION: SPECIFIC EXAMPLES

The first major post-World War II curricular innovation in medicine was that of Western Reserve University.[2] Begun in the mid-1950s and supported by the Commonwealth Fund, this became the model against which most subsequent curricular revisions were compared for the next two or three decades. It was the beginning of a significant effort in the United States to do something about the way in which medical students learned their trade. While there were many parts to this revision, one of the main reforms was in the teaching of basic science. Multidisciplinary student laboratories designed to accommodate basic sciences such as physiology and biochemistry, were incorporated in a comprehensive plan that was organized and monitored by relevant teaching committees. The basic sciences were taught in the context of interdisciplinary group learning about the various organ systems so as to promote their relevance to disease processes in patients. In addition, a presumably healthy family was assigned to each first year student, to be followed under supervision for at least two years. This sweeping curricular change had broad-based faculty support.

Other schools responded to this educational stimulus. The Stanford Medical School program was revised,[3] and some newer schools such as the University of Kentucky,[4] State University of New York (SUNY) at Stonybrook,[5] Michigan State University,[6] Pennsylvania State University,[7] and Brown University[8] adopted some innovations. These developments represented a nation-wide recognition of a need not only to increase the supply of American physicians but also to adapt their learning process to perceived community needs. The route taken reflected in large part the results of the widespread activity of research in medical education.

For example, at Stanford, where the institutional mission had been established with an emphasis on increasing its contribution to the quality and quantity of research-based academicians, medical school education was increased to five years. Teaching committees were established for each of seven curriculum segments. One segment, "Introduction to Clinical Medicine" provided the content and process for the transition from the basic sciences to the clinical years. A grant from the Russel Sage Foundation funded the addition of a behavioral science faculty member to each of the teaching committees. During the first three preclinical years, 50 percent of student time was labeled "free." This free time was initially defined as belonging to the students and was beyond the faculty's control. In view of the academically-oriented educational ambience, it was hoped that some of that free time would be used for research purposes. Among the reasons for the new program's short duration were departmental resentment over the loss of traditional control of curriculum, and the financial strain imposed on students by the five years of study. The original goal, however, of a highly academic educational program, with much opportunity for student autonomy, has persisted.

At Kentucky, a Department of Community Medicine (in lieu of the more usual Preventive Medicine) was established. Behavioral Sciences were departmentalized in similar fashion, and the curriculum was developed around quality of patient care. Stonybrook also instituted a Department of Humanities and Behavioral Science and did its best to integrate Medicine with Nursing and Allied Health Professions, Dental Medicine, Basic Health Sciences, and Social Welfare. These were all contained within a new administrative and architectural structure—the Health Sciences Center.

Michigan State University's College of Human Medicine began with the assumption that the existing basic science departments already serving a number of colleges, including Veterinary Medicine, would also relate to Human Medicine through new administrative links. The social sciences of anthropology, sociology, and psychology were included in the same fashion. As the curriculum developed, traditional lectures in the basic sciences were kept to a minimum by the use of an invention known as "focal problems."[9] In focal problems students learned basic science, pathophysiology, and clinical material in the context of small groups that studied simulated problems such as "chest pain," "high blood pressure," and "family planning." In the late 1960s, this initiative was a pioneering variant of the Western Reserve Committee arrangement. Now, in 1990, it is becoming fairly widespread under the rubric of "problem-based-learning." During the 1970s, Michigan State University added a College of Osteopathic Medicine with many of the same administrative arrangements as those characterizing the College of Human Medicine. This development, while politically instigated, had its serendipitous side: it provided an opportunity to assess the relationships between allopathic and osteopathic medicine, to ascertain the similarities and differences between the two professions, and to help diminish the destructive antipathy which in the past has characterized much of this interprofessional interaction. The two colleges continue to function as separate entities with a number of joint administrative and departmental arrangements. Many doubt that this dichotomy can continue indefinitely, and this academic setting could become a locus for working out the ways in which unification might some day transpire.

At Hershey Medical Center, Pennsylvania State University, separate departments of Humanities and of Behavioral Sciences were established. Their courses are required of all students, and some faculty members have made important contributions to the literature of humanities and behavioral science in medicine. Brown University, in getting on with its program in medical education, integrated its sequence with the final years of university preclinical education, and established a model for medical education as a continuum.

These instances of intense educational activity represent but a small sample of the many institutions involved in this remarkable response to an expressed public need for change in both the quality and quantity of those graduated from medical schools. I have cited those institutions with which I was personally familiar, either through direct involvement as faculty or administrator, in the context of participation in their accreditation site visits, or through various formalized relationships with their deans or other faculty leaders in relevant AAMC-related groups. Other institutions not mentioned here may well have been equally or even more noteworthy as innovators, and for their omission I apologize. I have simply tried to indicate the nature of some of the changes which occurred. It should also be noted that steadfast adherence to traditional educational patterns was the style of many existing institutions, and of a number of new schools as well.

55

THE TEACHING INSTITUTES OF THE AAMC: 1950s AND EARLY 1960s

Coincidentally with the curricular developments at Western Reserve in the 1950s and early 1960s, the AAMC exhibited a creative spurt of interest in educational issues and sponsored a series of Teaching Institutes. Not yet executive director, Ward Darley was a prominent member of the AAMC. In the planning stages for the institutes, a statement on the "Objectives of Undergraduate Medical Education"[10] appeared, and was first used in the Conference on Preventive Medicine in November 1952. At the request of the proposed institute's planning committee, a tentative draft that had been developed at the AAMC's central office was sent to each member of the Executive Council during the summer of 1951. A year later the draft had undergone six revisions; at the Preventive Medicine Teaching Institute, a seventh revision had been made, including suggestions from Western Reserve, and from the University of Colorado, where Ward Darley, having been dean of the medical school, was then president. The document comprising the work cited here was the eighth revision, and was still considered a "document under revision" open to comments and suggestions. This story is presented to reveal the difficulty experienced by the AAMC in coming to agreement on an issue which seemingly could have been entrusted to staff or a responsible committee.

Nonetheless, this document presages by more than a decade the principles which would become fundamental to much educational reform. For example:

[Undergraduate medical education] should not aim at presenting the complete, detailed, systematic body of knowledge concerning each and every medical and related discipline. Rather, it must provide the setting in which the student can learn fundamental principles applicable to the whole body of medical knowledge, establish habits of reasoned and critical judgment of evidence and experience, and develop an ability to use these principles and judgments wisely in solving problems of health and disease.

Undergraduate medical education cannot achieve these aims if the student is relegated to a passive role. It must provide incentive for active learning on the part of the student. This can best be done by giving him definite responsibility in real, day-to-day problems of health and disease, be carefully graded to the student's ability and experience and must be exercised under careful guidance by the faculty.

The document then goes on to list five aims, as follows:

1. To help the student acquire requisite knowledge;
2. To help the student establish essential habits;
3. To help the student achieve basic skills;

4. To help the student develop sound attitudes;
5. To help the student gain an understanding of professional and ethical principles.

That some AAMC leaders were clearly ahead of their time is clear from some of Dr. Darley's writings. For example, in 1959 he published a paper on the AAMC's objectives and program.[11] This paper describes in general the Teaching Institutes, and touches on medical school accreditation. In his description of the Liaison Committee, and its procedures, he states:

> The visiting teams represent the best collective thinking of the educators and the profession. The standards that are adhered to are quite general and are set up so as to provide an umbrella under which each school can use its own initiative in planning an effective curriculum. No attempt is made to dictate what should be taught or the number of hours a subject should require or to legislate regarding faculty, equipment or facilities. The visitors are free to use their judgment as to the nature and extent of any recommendations they may develop for the consideration of either the school being visited or the Liaison committee and its parent organizations. It is rare that the visitors' recommendations are not accepted by all concerned.[12]

In 1965 his speech at the Denver meeting of the AAMC was published.[13] This speech describes the AAMC's efforts to promote educational innovation. It includes several strong statements on research in medical education, and refers to collaborative efforts with George Miller. "One outcome of this Project was a series of seminars in which interested faculty could explore the factors involved in designing educational programs in accord with established concepts of learning theory." Since this was Darley's last address to the association as its leader, one must assume that his emphasis on medical education innovation and research reflected the association's emphasis during the time of his leadership.

Ward Darley had become executive director of the AAMC in 1957 and held that position until 1965. He had been present as a participant in 1953 in the first Teaching Institute.[14] With large representation from the faculties of many medical schools, discussions were wide-ranging and seem to have touched most of the educational issues then plaguing medical education. Controversy would seem to have been prominent in these meetings: for example, the research-teaching conflict was discussed. There were graphs in the write-up of the Pathology, Microbiology, Immunology, and Genetics Institute, showing that over 60 percent of both pathology and microbiology participants felt that good teaching depended on active participation in fundamental research, practical application thereof, and continued activity in both.[15] Between 50 and 60 percent of faculty felt that there was a shortage of teachers (microbiology and pathology) in their departments.[16] Serious conflict between teaching and research as ways of life did not emerge, however, with both microbiologists and pathologists identifying over 30 percent of their time as having been spent on teaching. There was a significant disaffection with the amount of research actually being done, with less than 20 percent of time actually spent in that activity, and nearly 35 percent being the amount desired.[17]

In 1955 an additional institute was held on Anatomy, Histology, Embryology and Anthropology. In 1956 and 1957, the institutes were designed as a pair on Evaluation of the Student, while the 1958 institute was on Clinical Teaching. A second institute on Clinical Teaching was held later in 1958.[18]

It is clear, then, that serious efforts were being expended by the AAMC on curriculum, with attention being paid to some of the most serious problems, and with results published in widely read journals. That these institutes were being held was common knowledge. With Dr. Darley as executive director of the AAMC it seemed clear that the organization was active in support of better education. With the AAMC involving faculty members in discussions such as these, it is not surprising that medical faculties talked about such issues, and that some became interested in possibilities of new programs and their opportunities for new kinds of pedagogy. Indeed, during this time the AAMC, not only through the publications of its executive director but through its sponsorship of such activities as the Teaching Institutes and specific programs of educational research, seemed to be seriously encouraging widespread reconsideration of the traditional modes of medical education.

ADMINISTRATIVE AND ACADEMIC ISSUES IN SUBSTITUTING THE NEW FOR THE TRADITIONAL TEACHING METHODS

The typical medical faculty member, whether M.D. or Ph.D., has undergone arduous and extended educational experience simply in quest of the doctoral degree. In either category, the primacy of research in the value system of science and medicine has been learned and accepted along with the necessity for research excellence to insure academic success. Certainly by the time a position of significant status and power has been attained, the validity of this paradigm has become self-evident. Students, residents, and younger faculty are advised to follow in these footsteps, and are quite likely warned against being seduced by the temptations of or administrative pressure toward increased involvement in teaching. Furthermore, it is unlikely that specific attention had been paid in their educational experiences to learning pedagogical skills. It is simply assumed that qualifications as teachers automatically result from the acquisition of knowledge and from clinical experience and research accomplishment. It is generally felt by science and medical faculty that pedagogy as studied, practiced, and learned in colleges of education is "soft," encumbered with irrelevant jargon, and unlikely to be useful in scientific or medical settings. Partly from such a nearly universal set of attitudes, built-in prejudice against and resistance to change in educational form, content, or method is the norm.

When the amount of time and effort needed to put such a modern educational model into effect becomes clear, the reaction may even become disturbingly antagonistic. For example, at Michigan State, where a variant of problem-based learning had become college policy, one basic science department flatly refused to participate, saying that students would learn their field only by the usual departmental lecture route—the faculty was far too busy to become involved in a time-consuming educational effort of unproven merit. While this position failed to thwart the program, it did force some unwanted educational and administrative compromises.

Particularly at the preclinical level, the traditional medical school course is arranged as though the main preparation for a career in medicine is the accumulation of knowledge. Memorization of incredible amounts of factual material can generate a kind of cold cynicism which seems to be part of what the public today reluctantly experiences from many of its technically expert physicians. Furthermore, the intense effort to concentrate on the entire biomedical subject matter eliminates time for such important subjects as medical ethics and other aspects of the humanities. Free time for other aspects of self development is also virtually nonexistent.

Another serious matter at all levels of education is the complexity of evaluation. From the faculty's standpoint, the simplest, most direct, and most easily managed form of testing is a multiple choice instrument developed by an outside agency such as the National Board of Medical Examiners (NBME). Such a program relieves them of the time-consuming and tedious process of developing such examinations themselves, of testing the validity of their questions, and of establishing guidelines for academic success. Furthermore, since many faculty members participate in the production of NBME questions, they put in their time at the relevant sessions under the exceedingly good guidance of the expert evaluation staff of that organization. So-called "shelf examinations" can be obtained from the NBME for use as interim testing tools during the course of study. It is possible to set up a curriculum with minimal faculty involvement, therefore, in which the vast majority of the evaluation process is handled by outsiders. Some National Board issues, the division of the examination into three parts, the dichotomy resulting between basic science and clinical medicine by the insertion of Part I at the end of the second year, and the failure of the NBME's effort to eliminate Part I have been described in chapter 2. While the normal National Board sequence is not incompatible with curricular reform to promote educational continuum it can, and sometimes does, significantly impair its effectiveness.

During the 1960s and 1970s, a period of great growth and change in medical education, most medical faculties included some individuals who believed in the need for curricular change, read the educational research literature and, indeed, may have been involved in innovative projects within traditional teaching programs. I accepted the offer of the deanship at Michigan State as my response to the ferment of the times and because of the opportunity to accomplish important new things there. While the existing basic science departments were good in research and traditional in their educational styles, the big recruitment opportunity was in filling the new positions made available in the science departments, and in the establishment of a new clinical faculty. Selective recruitment gradually resulted in a faculty in favor of exploiting the opportunities in this setting for curricular innovation. While considerable strife ensued, much constructive change occurred and, to a surprising extent, persists.

On the other hand, some universities that newly undertook medical education opted for an emphasis on research and the development of academic medical centers, with curricular innovation a less prominent objective. In any case, the 1960s and 1970s were years of significant expansion of medical school enrollments, both in enlarged existing schools and new institutions. Considerable conflict arose between the contrasting educational factions, not only in the schools themselves but also within the AAMC and in the LCME, whose accreditation decisions were critical in fashioning the results of this process. On the one hand were the traditionalists, with their firm roots in basic research and the corollary belief in the sanctity of quality which was defined for faculty as research success and for students as achievement in academic grades and performance in the laboratory. On the other hand were those deeply concerned about the negative impact of "overspecialization," the spiraling cost of medical care, and the dulling and antihumanistic effect on students of countless hours of lectures. These faculty members tended to be excited by the new educational possibilities emerging from pedagogical research, relevant investigations in the behavioral sciences, and the development of the new area of the humanities in medicine.

This period was also a time of proliferation of exciting and significant discoveries in such fields as immunology, transplantation, and invasive and diagnostic medicine. NIH and foundation-based funding for research and research-training escalated. With increased funding simultaneously appearing for biomedical research and for programs in educational research, community medicine, and medical humanities, each camp became increasingly well-armed. All of this was happening during the post-Coggeshall period of the AAMC, whose staff expanded in an effort to keep up with these protean and conflicting developments within its member institutions. As the era proceeded, the ambient tumult reflected the student and social unrest coincident with the Johnson administration and the Vietnam War.

It was indeed a fascinating period, similar in some ways to the Progressive Era. Riska calls attention to this analogy: "There have been at least two major periods of social reform in 20th century American social history: one was the Progressive Era at the turn of the century (1890–1914) and the last was the era of the Great Society (1960–1967)."[19] She feels it no accident that two periods of medical education reform occurred in these two times of recognition of need for major change in the correction of deficiencies in American society. She goes on to wonder whether the reforms of the Great Society can continue in a period of sustained political and social conservatism.

While the modification of the style of student learning by substitution of problem-based learning for the traditional lecture mode has perhaps received the most attention from medical faculties, other developments have been of comparable significance. These include the inclusion of medical humanities in curriculum content and medical practice, student-generated concern for medical care for the poor, community hospitals as sites for required clinical education, and the advent of the discipline of family practice.

THE MEDICAL HUMANITIES AND THE BEHAVIORAL AND SOCIAL SCIENCES

Ever since Abraham Flexner, scholars have written about the essential nature of the humanities in the education of physicians. He stated in his report, for example:

Such enlargement of the physician's horizon is otherwise important, for scientific progress has greatly modified his ethical responsibility. His relation was formerly to his patient ... at most to the patient's family; and it was almost altogether remedial.... But the physician's function is fast becoming social and preventive, rather than individual and curative. Upon him society relies to ascertain, and through measures essentially educational to enforce, the conditions that prevent disease and make positively for physical and moral well-being. It goes without saying that this type of doctor is first of all an educated man.[20]

While few really dispute these sorts of statements, they do deny that valuable time in medical school should be given over to philosophers and other "soft-minded" teachers, when there is so much "hard" material to be learned.

The idea that it is essential for physicians to understand something about ethical and moral reflection, to have studied some relevant literature, and to be aware of some of the limitations of modern medicine is not universally felt by practicing physicians or medical educators. The idea of the physician as benign paternalist always acting in the best interest of his patient, issuing "orders" which the good patient must obey, and rarely allowing his patient's querulous-

61

ness to stand in the way of what the doctor knows to be best for him, has been firmly ingrained into Western medicine. While cure of illness and relief of suffering have ever been the avowed primary objectives of patient care, it almost seems that prevention of death, the ultimate symbol of medical failure, has assumed the highest position on the value scale in this era of high-technology medicine. With many high-tech tools, the fruits of scientific research, and advances in engineering, it almost seems that application of these research-generated modalities is attempting to fulfill Gates' semi-religious predictions for the all-encompassing success of this sanctified activity.[21]

In seeking guidance for indications for the moral course vis-à-vis selective use of technology in terminal illness, physicians had long respected the Catholic distinction between ordinary and extraordinary care. It was the 1970s case of Karen Quinlan, however, and the ruling of the New Jersey Supreme Court supporting the parents' wishes that artificial respiratory support be discontinued in the case of their daughter's permanent vegetative state, which really provided the impetus for the ensuing growth spurt of medical ethics. Beginning with a group of ministers associated with medical schools, the Society for Health and Human Values was formed by a few deans, medical faculty members, and clergy and philosophers interested in the subject. Leadership emerged from a number of medical schools including Hershey Medical Center of Pennsylvania State University, Georgetown University, SUNY at Stonybrook, and Michigan State University. Through a national program of site visits to medical schools and the emergence of federal funding opportunities from the National Endowment for the Humanities, medical humanities programs—sometimes with departmental or divisional status—were established so that somewhere in the teaching programs of most institutions there is significant representation of ethics, philosophy, and literature as it relates to medicine.

Independent of the Society of Health and Human Values, but including some of the same interested faculty, the Hastings Center was developed. This establishment, with a distinguished board of directors and physical headquarters at Briarcliff Manor, New York, is both the publisher of the quarterly *Hastings Center Report*, and a center for advanced study in the humanities related to health and medicine.

It should be noted that this development has occurred almost simultaneously with the expansion of the role of the behavioral and social sciences in medical education, and the growth of its related national group, the Association for the Behavioral Sciences in Medical Education (ABSAME). It likewise developed as a corollary to the recognition in some quarters of the essential nature of behavioral and social science thought and research to the history and development of modern medicine, and to the vital nature of its content to education for the health professions.

To a large degree, the common ground for both social scientists and humanists has to do with respect for and understanding of the nature of the human person. Through social science we learn about such features of man as the relevance of ethnicity, social class, and environmental influence on status, personality, and reaction to stress and illness. Conclusions in these fields are derived through research in psychology, anthropology, and sociology, and are employed by informed teachers in such applications as doctor-patient interaction as they work with students during their clinical years. Some understanding of research methodology in the social sciences, therefore, is important to the educated physician.

Rather than through research in its usual sense, the process through which ethical analysis of human dilemmas is achieved is characterized by the rigorous application of rules of logic and philosophical analysis to the situation at hand. Classical philosophical literature of the Western world is replete with authors of immense stature such as Plato, Immanuel Kant, and John Stuart Mill.[22] Leading modern philosophers interested in medicine include Joseph Fletcher, Tristram Englehardt, Daniel Callahan, Alasdair MacIntyre, John Rawls, and Robert Veatch.[23]

The field is huge and includes such areas of involvement as ethics in research, moral issues in abortion, genetic counseling, behavior control, and discontinuation of life support systems. Most of the focus is on the rights of the individual patient based on the notion of autonomy, and expresses itself in the form of the doctrine of informed consent. While informed consent has been applied as a feature of those dilemmas indigenous to tertiary care, thinking has now extended its application to the office practice of primary care.[24] In ethical terms, the patient is the critical partner in the patient-physician transaction to whom the physician, except in the most extreme circumstance, can do nothing without consent. The degree to which consent is explicit varies with the situation, but it is now possible that physicians may be legally liable if it can be shown that the patient's right to such autonomy has been violated.

The issues encompassing the fields of humanities and social sciences in medicine are strikingly relevant to much of the current dissonance between medicine and the public. The alleged inability of physicians to listen to patients, their sometimes seemingly fanatic reliance on life-support systems in the face of opposition from patient or family, revealed fraud in the conduct of research, and the ever-increasing distrust between the legal and medical professions emanating from the malpractice impasse are among the situations, so important to the public and physicians alike, which are within the purview of the humanities and social sciences.

These subjects usually appear in the medical school curricula during the preclinical years either in lecture form, as learning objectives in problem-based learning, or in the context of special "ethics rounds" in a teaching hospital. It is rare, however, for ethical issues to be stressed either in the usual context of the clinical clerkship, in grand rounds, or in the day-to-day experiences of patient care delivered by faculty in the wards or in the clinics. Indeed, this was strongly emphasized by one of our most prominent and influential medical ethicists at a recent AAMC annual meeting.[25] Without strong reinforcement at the clinical level, and without the fervor comparable to that accorded biochemical relevance, little lasting impact on students or residents can be expected. A beginning has been made, and the LCME now mentions medical ethics and behavioral sciences in its guidelines for accreditation, but great change in the thinking or behavior of graduates has yet to be observed. In the community in which I now live, practice is generally in the tradition of benign paternalism: doing what is thought best for patients, and tending to resent overt emphasis on, or discussion of, autonomy, informed consent, or the medical contribution to the problem of malpractice and medical liability. There has not been a serious effort to establish a hospital ethics committee, and the malpractice issue is ascribed to the predatory nature of the legal profession. I feel certain that this represents the practice mode and prevailing attitude of the vast majority of American physicians.

RESPONSE TO PUBLIC PRESSURE: FAMILY PRACTICE— A NEW POWER BASE FOR PRIMARY CARE

While the initiative for the inclusion of medical humanities in the structure and function of medical schools originated in the academic community, the impetus for emphasizing primary care during the educational process stemmed largely from extramural pressure. General practitioners, long the mainstay of American medical care, had been diminishing in numbers and prestige since World War II. The sharp turn toward specialization in the career choices of medical school graduates had moved the responsibility for providing primary care to internists, pediatricians, obstetricians, and even surgeons. Evidence was accumulating that delivering such care was of secondary interest to physicians who were trained as specialists, that it seemed to lack the personal touch of the "old time family doctor," and that it was more dependent on the laboratory—and hence more costly—than it had previously been. Beginning in the mid-1960s the force for reestablishing the respectability of family medicine was exerted by the general public, the media, the AMA, and federal and state governments. It seems fair to state that medical schools, particularly the private prestigious ones, and the AAMC had little real interest in this development. Their attitude was that specialists were generally capable of delivering primary care, that the movement was generally anti-intellectual, and that family medicine was an activity without either a research base or an academic tradition on which to establish a viable academic discipline.

Among the important steps in the development of family practice was the 1966 AMA-appointed commission chaired by John Millis, then president of Case-Western Reserve University.[26] The commission attributed the decline of general practice in part to the recent change of student career choice during medical school. It stated the need for appropriate changes in educational programs to reverse this tendency. A committee spawned by the AMA at about the same time, and chaired by William Willard, dean of the University of Kentucky Medical School, developed the idea of Family Practice as a necessary medical specialty with specific educational features, and labeled the proposed specialist in primary care the Family Physician.[27] It emphasized the need for a major change in medical education to accompany the described developments. In its journal *GP*, the American Academy of General Practice published a report in the same year which formulated the general core content for family medicine. The idea of the family practice residency as the requisite graduate training program was getting under way.[28]

In one of the early textbooks on Family Medicine, John Geyman emphasized the deleterious effect on training for primary care in medical schools resulting from de-emphasis of general practice and primary care in favor of exposure entirely to the specialist model.[29] While many students entered medical school with general practice as their ultimate goal of postgraduation activity, most chose before graduation to specialize. He also noted the societal enthusiasm for technical procedures and the increasing concentration of knowledge in narrow areas. Students, in his view, saw these as more important than the care of common clinical problems or the uniqueness of the patient as a person. He also felt that the predominance of solo practice among general practitioners served as an additional deterrent to the selection of primary care as a career.

Graduate training, likewise, was not thriving. While during the 1950s and 1960s there were a few two-year general practice residencies in community hospitals, the annual national tally of residents numbered but 400 to 500. By contrast, the number of specialty residents soared from 20,000 in 1960 to over 35,000 in 1968; by the late 1960s only one physician in five was in general practice.

In any case, a movement was underway, and family practice was in the process of becoming a specialty. In 1971 the American Academy of General Practice became the American Academy of Family Physicians. It has continued to play a vital role in the development of the field, especially in the facilitation of education programs and through liaison with other specialities and various levels of government. Since 1969 the American Board of Family Practice has been responsible for development and implementation of certification and recertification procedures, and is responsible for the maintenance of standards. Examinations have been given annually since 1970. There are now over 32,000 diplomates of the Board, and over 55,000 members of the Academy of Family Physicians. Their peak ages are 34 and 59 years, and over the next ten years will become the youngest of the specialties.

Graduate training programs in family practice now exist in about 75 percent of today's medical schools; 10.9 percent have no known plans for such programs; there are divisions of family practice in 8.7 percent, and planning is proceeding in 0.7 percent.[30] In July 1984 there were 375 accredited programs, up from 15 in 1969. Faculty recruitment, however, has been difficult because of the lack of a family practice tradition in academic medicine. In 1971–72, the number of family practice faculty was 82; in 1983–84 it was up to 1148.[31] The specialty of family practice, then, has been established with its own academy and methodology for the maintenance of standards of medical practice which have largely to do with primary care and the way it is practiced.

Established, but not yet truly secure; funding for family practice has thus far been initiated by governmental or other ad hoc temporary grants or tentative arrangements, and sometimes through initiatives by interested hospitals. Geyman lists four main sources of funding; (1) patient-care revenue; (2) the contributions of participating hospitals; (3) state funding, often on a capitation basis; and (4) grants from federal, foundation, or other sources.[32] He considers the grants option to be "soft," since such funds are usually limited to getting programs started. Patient-care revenue, once established, is dependable, but should not cover more than half of total program costs. The contribution of the host hospital must therefore provide a solid floor of funding for the residency program. It should be noted that it is the "hospital" which is cited as the most important source of support, rather than the medical school or university.

The costs of family practice residencies are substantial, and average over $50,000 per resident, including the salary of over $17,000 and prorated costs for faculty, staff, teaching materials, operational costs of the Family Practice Center and related expenses.[33] Each program, then, must be fiscally justified on the basis of the hospitals' financial condition. The number of family practice residencies in the United States plateaued at 386 in 1981, and in 1984 had fallen to 384.[34] This level of residency places accommodated about 13 percent of the 16,000 medical school graduates each year. Since many advocate that family practice residencies should be able to accommodate at least 25 percent of American medical graduates, there is concern about the health of this movement. With the enthusiastic support of some state legislatures now having waned, and with specialist advocates in such fields as internal medicine and pediatrics averring that family practice may have outrun its usefulness, there is evidence of lagging momentum. Hospitals, furthermore, are experiencing increasing financial difficulties, and the abolition or diminution in size or quality of a residency could be one way out of such a predicament.

Geyman reflects the need for the new specialty of family practice to develop an appropriate field of research.[35] He summarizes research publications in the *Journal of Family Practice* between 1974 and 1982. Observational research leads the list, with case studies, reviews, opinion, methods, and experimental investigation in decreasing measure. Contrary to the situation with the traditional medical specialties whose research is usually based in the "exact" biological sciences, investigation attributable to family practice appears to derive more from the social and behavioral sciences and humanities, and generally reflects the "holistic" interests of this new discipline. Just as it has been hard for medical faculties to accept social scientists and humanists as academic colleagues, so is it the case with family medicine. Partly for this reason, the acceptance of this new discipline by the establishment is tentative. The unavailability of a significant number of academically trained family physicians accustomed to the teaching and research responsibilities of medical academe inhibits departmental growth with experienced faculty. The long-term future of family medicine in the medical school faculty, therefore, is still uncertain. It seems particularly vulnerable now, with the current period of generally restricted medical school financing, and with the lowered volume of specific federal grant support for family medicine programs.

With primary care at the heart of the nation's medical care problem, it would be a pity if the main academic initiative with the goal of doing something constructive in this area were seriously inhibited by its ultimate inability to become "one of the academic boys." It seems clear that departments or divisions of family practice do not flourish within the traditional academic medical center and it could well be true that such a deviation from a center's central mission is a needlessly distracting enterprise. Were such to be recognized as a valid state of affairs, newer and more community-oriented institutions should be encouraged to concentrate on primary care and family practice and should be absolved from the need to compete in the more traditional academic medical fields. (This will be further discussed in chapter 5, as the issue of accreditation is pursued in depth.) The potential for family practice to collaborate with such colleagues as social scientists, economists, demographers, and public health departments is promising, and could provide the means by which real leadership could emerge in research geared to such problems as access, health delivery to the rural poor, and imaginative ways to more effectively provide health education for communities whose culture is out of phase with our own.

In schools with which I am most familiar, I have been highly impressed with the quality of the performance of family medicine throughout the continuum of medical education. The Family Practice Department at Michigan State administers the early experiences for third-year students in clinical medicine, and shares with other clinical departments teaching in the closed-circuit television patient interviewing program. There are two family practice residencies in the Lansing area related to the department. At Mercer, the Department of Family Medicine, the largest full-time department in the school, conceived and manages the entire statewide preceptorship program, experienced by all students throughout their entire course of study, and in which they become intensely aware of the problems and promise of rural primary care.

In my opinion, the addition of the Family Practice residency to the constellation of graduate training programs is impressive. Based in self-contained practices and with offices either within or adjacent to hospitals, these programs provide both in-house experiences equivalent to those of rotating internships, and three-year ambulatory care programs in the context of continuing care in defined populations of patients. The opportunity exists, then, both for intensive experience in the primary care mode for patients regardless of age or disease category, and to learn the role and expertise of the various specialties in the provision of comprehensive care. Furthermore, a smaller, semirural hospital, unable to support a traditional specialty training program, is sometimes in a position to maintain a family practice residency with many of the traditional residency-related benefits to in-patient care.

Finally, I have been impressed with the quality and dedication of the new family physicians I have known. They tend to practice in group settings, to have well-equipped offices, and to be well informed in the multitude of areas with which this branch of medicine must be familiar. They seem to work comfortably in community hospitals with specialists, refer patients to them, and enjoy their respect. Certainly for the middle class, and for those adequately covered with health insurance, the addition of family practice to the medical community should do much to solve the primary care problem.

The notion that the addition of specific competence in the field of primary and ambulatory care to the available mix of practicing physicians will solve the problem of accessibility to the poor urban and rural underserved, however, is clearly not true. For example, the issue of the financial burden on the local hospital caused by the necessity to care for indigent patients was discussed at a recent meeting of the county medical society in my semi-rural community. Local state legislators, the health department director, the hospital administrator, and interested local industrialists all expressed empathy for the plight of the poor. Their sympathy extended not only to the fundamentally needy but to those with parttime employment and the resulting lack of hospital insurance. This meeting seemed to recognize not only the serious need for supplementation of Medicare and Medicaid funding, but also for expanding public funding beyond the rigid definitions of beneficiaries of these two government programs. It occurred to me that this medical society meeting could presage an avenue through which the medical private sector could cooperate with government and other community agencies in a desperately needed public dialogue.

For the first time in recent years, the 1989 AAMC Annual Meeting featured a major program on rural health, with Sen. Robert Dole as keynote speaker. The main speech by Kevin Fickenscher was a challenge to the academic community to become seriously involved in education for and research in rural health care problems, and to be aware that effecting real improvement in rural health involves not only provision of good medical care, but also in rebuilding the infrastructure of rural communities.[36] Fickenscher said, for example, " . . . rural people who represent 25 percent of the nation's population deserve access to the same level and quality of health care as their urban counterparts." It could be that a new interest on the part of the federal government and the AAMC in rural health is in the making.

At the 1990 spring meeting of the AAMC's Council of Deans, the dean and provost for medical affairs at Mercer University School of Medicine spoke on the subject of "Primary Care Education and Service: The Role of Medical Schools."[37] This presentation was an elegant statement of the need for more primary care physicians, particularly in rural areas, and the necessity for medical schools consciously to increase their emphasis on primary care experiences and to increase applicants' motivation for primary care in priorities favoring admission. He made clear, however, the hazard of allowing legislators to assume that the establishment of medical school-based family practice programs will automatically solve the rural access problem. While medical education is fundamental to the way in which physicians think, behave, and make career choices, dollars for education must not be permitted to absolve society of its responsibilities for the public's health care.

After this talk, the meeting broke up into small discussion groups. The group of deans in which I participated expressed little enthusiasm for taking on the additional responsibility of primary care teaching or programs. In the current period of budget struggles and steadily decreasing success by investigators in obtaining funding for their NIH research grants, primary care did not emerge as a high priority item.

Thus, while the AAMC's new interest in rural health and primary care is encouraging, it would seem that what is needed in this day of uncertainty in medical school financing may be a major governmental program to offset the skewed nature of the institutional response to NIH-funded research, and to provide money for effective education in primary care, relevant health care research, and other activities designed to modify the total spectrum of graduates of American medical schools in a way that will more constructively meet the nation's health care needs.

MORE PUBLIC PRESSURE: AFFIRMATIVE ACTION AND
MEDICAL CARE FOR THE POOR

On my arrival at Michigan State in 1964, while there was specific land-grant–oriented interest in health care for rural Michigan, there was no notion that enrollment of women or minorities was a high priority in our proposed new medical school. As in most American institutions, this priority emerged as a result of the general ground-swell of student activism as part and parcel of the civil rights movement that peaked toward the end of the 1960s. With specific legislative funding, the university had established a College of Urban Affairs whose purposes included increasing minority student enrollment and developing curriculum and research activities in minority affairs. The new medical school was one of its early targets, and a visit to my office by two intensely dedicated black students stands out as one of the more memorable surprises of my deanship. Within a remarkably short time, and with funding from this new college, we had developed a medical preparatory program for minority students. Their enrollment soon escalated to the point that they comprised up to 25 percent of each class. One outcome of the civil rights movement on national policy vis-à-vis the universities was affirmative action, with enforced requirements that minorities be added in considerable number to student bodies, faculties, and all staff levels on pain of forfeiture of all types of federal funding. The AAMC developed its staff to include Minority Affairs, and the concept of a medical school student body with but token Blacks, Latinos, or Native Americans began to disappear. It has been my observation that students, whatever their racial origins, have by and large been pleased with this new state of affairs, and that the scope and interests of medical education have benefited. It would be fatuous to claim that there have not been problems, but I think that our response to this social development has by and large been exemplary.

This time of pro-minority social action, during the late 1960s when the deep concern of the Johnson administration for the poor had not yet been driven off the nation's agenda by the excruciating costs of the Vietnam conflict, reflected itself in participation by some medical schools in War on Poverty programs such as community health centers. Grants were available from the Office of Economic Opportunity (OEO), with guidelines for such community-based programs having been written by government staff. One of the more famous of such efforts was that developed at Tufts Medical School in Boston.[38] Although we did not as yet have students in clinical training at Michigan State, we successfully applied to OEO for the first rural community health center, in collaboration with the state health department. It is still in operation, supported by the community with all federal funding long since discontinued. These programs included not only medical care, but nursing, pharmacy, home health, mental health, and health education. They were idealistic in the extreme and very costly, but had Vietnam not interfered, some sort of permanent arrangement could well have emerged. Indeed, had war not thwarted this national program in which a number of medical schools were involved in demonstrations of academic-community partnership, it is entirely possible that the depth of today's access and primary care problems might have been largely prevented.

Another initiative of the time was the Heart, Cancer and Stroke Program, which evolved into Regional Medical Programs. These were national incentives to lure academic medical centers out of their home bases to assume educational and care responsibilities for other communities in their regions. Thus, through administrative links, personnel sharing, and diffusion of technology, the academic medical center would have arms out to the rest of the region. Grants obtained by the medical schools, or in collaboration with one or more nearby communities, specified the development of "coopera-tive arrangements" not only between the medical school and its community extensions, but also between the various medical schools in the state or region. Hence, in the Philadelphia area, the Delaware Valley Regional Medical Program developed, and in Michigan this initiative forced the three state universities with medical schools into their first truly amicable health-oriented coop-erative arrangement. The overall purpose of this national program was to formalize an effective extension of the influence of the aca-demic medical centers into their regions to spread their influence not only in medical care but in undergraduate and graduate health education as well.

I have mentioned these initiatives of the early years of the Johnson administration as fond recollection of the excitement with which many of us implemented some of the initiatives floated by the federal government as it undertook to bring reality to the concept of the "Great Society." While some of the products of this national effort remain, the majority lost impetus as funds were withdrawn to implement our Vietnamese policies. Had the failure of these poli-cies not forced Johnson's retirement from the upcoming 1968 presi-dential race leaving the war to continue under a conservative ad-ministration with substitution of a new caution-ridden national mood, there is no telling where medical education would now find itself.

A few years later during the Nixon administration, the benefici-aries of affirmative action, now responding to the feministic pres-sure of the day, began to emphasize women as well as racial minori-ties. It should be noted that affirmative action's new emphasis on the right of women to be employed and enrolled on a par with men was essentially the result of a middle-class movement. Minority groups, for example, had long since felt the injustice of Medicaid's policy of requiring poor women to be employed in order to receive benefits for their children; such women would have liked nothing better than to enjoy the right of middle-class mothers to care for their children at home.

At the medical school level, this meant that women should no longer be discriminated against during the admission process, and that every effort should be made to include women as well as minorities as high priority candidates in faculty recruitment. Issues of potentially interrupted careers because of marriage and pregnancy would no longer be valid negative criteria. Women would no longer be given differential treatment as students in the examination of male patients during their clinical training. With criteria for admission of women identical with those for men, there developed a huge influx of women, who were often better qualified and better prepared than their male counterparts. One year, our director of admissions at Michigan State told me that it was almost discriminatory against women to admit any men at all! While this was not intended as a serious comment, it has been remarkable to notice the extent to which women, often with unusual backgrounds in other professions, health-related or not, have assumed leadership in student bodies, and become truly outstanding graduates. Even the most chauvinistic of male faculty members appear to have yielded to the stimulating effect of students with both sexes nearly equally represented.

THE CURRENT ERA: APPARENT SCARCITY OF RESOURCES

With the explosion of available funds and the excitement of the Johnson years long since passed, American medical education has lowered its aspirations in accord with the public expression of expectations. As public interest in health care for the poor lost urgency, medical centers, while performing as required to provide minimum care to acutely ill indigents, have lost interest in experimental health care demonstrations. Instead, they have quite understandably become basically concerned for their own survival. Instead of exhorting clinical faculty to engage in health care research for which there is presently little in the way of funding sources, deans urge their clinicians to spend ever-increasing time with patients so as to maintain and augment their incomes and to provide, through medical practice plans, needed revenue for the medical centers themselves. With the emphasis on the paying patient and high technology, the students' role models, rather than emphasizing care for the disadvantaged, are instead concerned for literate clients able to pay the high costs of their own care. The acceptable priorities are entirely clear to medical students and house officers alike.

There has been a striking rise in the incidence of spectacular surgery, with such events as the recent tour de force of triple transplantation of liver, heart, and kidney a topic of widespread media attention. Rural medical care hardly generates the enthusiastic public accolades with which the more glamorous medical accomplishments are celebrated. Particularly distressing are the ways in which the public is sometimes manipulated to raise money for such patients' hospitalizations and to pay the huge fees these procedures may entail. In spite of the almost desperate danger of American medicine being engulfed by its own extravagances, it must surely be counterproductive for some of our leading academic medical centers to provide such examples under the guise of humanistic medical progress in the best interest of the public.

Though the years of conservative government have presided over a sharp decrease—or even elimination—of funds for socially-oriented aspects of education for health care, the NIH budget has continued to rise, although not usually to the degree that the academic community deems appropriate. The 1990 administration-authorized budget is $7,638 billion.[39] Research funding, therefore, remains the major extramural source of support for American academic medicine.

NOTES

1. George Miller, et al., *Teaching and Learning in Medical School* (Cambridge: Harvard University Press, Commonwealth Fund, 1961).
2. J. T. Wearn, et al., "Reports on Experiments in Medical Education," *Journal of Medical Education* 31 (1956): 515–65. It is to be noted that the Commonwealth Fund was heavily involved in a number of curricular innovations. These are described in the excellent history of the fund by A. McGehee Harvey and Susan L. Abrams, *For the Welfare of Mankind; The Commonwealth Fund and American Medicine* (Baltimore: The Johns Hopkins University Press, 1986).
3. L. M. Stowe, "The Stanford Plan, an Educational Continuum for Medicine," *Journal of Medical Education* 34 (1959): 1059–69.
4. B. B. Baughman, "The Beginning of the Medical School of the University of Kentucky; the Political and Scientific Background; Louisville, 1979," *Journal of the Kentucky Medical Association* 77 (1979): 525–28.
5. E. D. Pellegrino, "State University of New York at Stony Brook Health Sciences Center," in *The Case Histories of Ten New Medical Schools*, ed. V. W. Lippard and E. F. Purcell (New York: The Josiah Macy Fr., Foundation, 1972), 241–95.
6. A. D. Hunt, "Michigan State University, College of Human Medicine," in *The Case Histories of Ten New Medical Schools*, ed. V. W. Lippard and E. F. Purcell (New York: The Josiah Macy Fr., Foundation, 1972), 167–208.
7. G. T. Harrell, "The Pennsylvania State University, The Milton S. Hershey Medical Center," in *The Case Histories of Ten New Medical Schools*, ed. V. W. Lippard and E. F. Purcell (New York: The Josiah Macy Fr., Foundation, 1972), 331–79.
8. P. M. Galetti, "Brown University; Division of Biological and Medical Sciences," in *The Case Histories of Ten New Medical Schools*, ed. V. W.

Lippard and E. F. Purcell (New York: The Josiah Macy Fr., Foundation, 1972), 33–84.

9. P. O. Ways, G. Loftus, and J. M. Jones, "Focal Problem Teaching in Medical Education," *Journal of Medical Education* 48 (1973): 565–71.

10. "The Objectives of Undergraduate Medical Education," *Journal of Medical Education* 28, no. 3 (1953): 57–59.

11. Ward Darley, "The Association of American Medical Colleges: Its Objectives and Program," *Journal of Medical Education* 34, no. 8 (1959): 814–18.

12. Ibid., 817.

13. Ward Darley, "AAMC Milestones in Raising the Standards of Medical Education," *Journal of Medical Education* 40, no. 4 (1965): 321–27.

14. As planned in 1953, these events were listed as follows: Institutes for the teaching of Physiology, Biochemistry and Pharmacology (1953); Pathology, Microbiology, Immunology and Genetics (1954); Anatomy, Histology, Embryology and Anthropology (1955); Medical Ecology (1956); Clinical Teaching, including the Internship (1957); and Specialty Training and the Continuing Education of the Physician (1958).

15. "The Teaching of Pathology, Microbiology, Immunology, Genetics, Report of the Second Teaching Institute, October 10–15, 1954," Part 2, *Journal of Medical Education* 30, no. 9 (1955): 91.

16. Ibid., 109.

17. Ibid., 115.

18. "The Teaching of Physiology, Biochemistry, Pharmacology; Report of the First Teaching Institute, AAMC, Atlantic City, October 19–23, 1953," *Journal of Medical Education* 29, no. 7 (1964) (in two parts); "The Teaching of Anatomy and Anthropology in Medical Education, AAMC, Swampscott, Mass., October 18–22, 1955," *Journal of Medical Education* 31, no. 10 (1956) (in two parts); "The Ecology of the Medical Student. Report of the Fifth Teaching Institute, AAMC, Atlantic City, N.J., October 15–19, 1957," *Journal of Medical Education* 33, no. 10 (1958); "Report of The First Institute on Clinical Teaching, Swampscott, Mass., October 7 to 11, 1958," *Association of American Medical Colleges,*, 1959; "Report of the Second Institute on Clinical Teaching, Report of the Seventh Institute, AAMC, Chicago, Ill., October 27–31, 1959, *Journal of Medical Education* 36, no. 4 (1961); and "Medical Education and Medical Care, Report of the Eighth Teaching Institute, AAMC, Hollywood Beach, Florida, November 1–3, 1960, *Journal of Medical Education* 36, no. 12 (1961).

19. Elianne Riska, "Social Reform and Reform in Medical Education," in *Marching to a Different Drummer, Medical Education Since 1960,* ed. A. D. Hunt and L. E. Weeks (East Lansing: Michigan State University Foundation, with support from the W. K. Kellogg Foundation, 1979), 340–56.

20. Abraham Flexner, *Medical Education in the United States and Canada; A Report to the Carnegie Foundation for the Advancement of Teaching,* Bulletin Number Four (Boston: D. P. Updike, The Merrymount Press, Boston, 1910).

21. Frederick Gates, "Memoirs of Frederick T. Gates," *American Heritage* 6, no. 3 (1955): 73–74.

22. Plato, *The Republic;* Immanuel Kant, *Groundwork of The Metaphysic*

of Morals, trans. H. J. Paton (New York: Harper and Row, 1964); John Stuart Mill, *Utilitarianism* (Indianapolis: Bobbs-Merrill, 1957).

23. Joseph Fletcher, *Morals and Medicine* (Boston: Beacon Press, 1954); H. Tristram Englehardt, Jr. and Daniel Callahan, *Science, Ethics and Medicine* (Hastings on Hudson, N.Y.: Institute of Society, Ethics and the Life Sciences, 1976); Alasdair MacIntyre, *A Short History of Ethics* (New York: Macmillan, 1966); John Rawls, *A Theory of Justice* (Cambridge: Harvard University Press, 1971); Robert M. Veatch, *Case Studies in Medical Ethics* (Cambridge: Harvard University Press, 1977); T. L. Beauchamp and J. F. Childress, *Principles of Biomedical Ethics* (New York: Oxford University Press, 1989; and C. M. Culver, et al., "Basic Curricular Goals in Medical Ethics," *N.E.J.M.* 312 (1985): 253–56.

24. Howard Brody, "Transparency: Informed Consent in Primary Care," *Hastings Center Report* 19, no. 5 (1989): 5–9.

25. A. P. Jonsen, "Leadership in Meeting Ethical Challenges," *Journal of Medical Education* 62, no. 2 (1987): 95–99.

26. *The Graduate Education of Physicians*, report of the Citizen's Commission on Graduate Medical Education (Millis Commission) (Chicago: American Medical Association, 1966).

27. *Meeting the Challenge of Family Practice,* report of the Ad Hoc Committee on Education for Family Practice of the Council on Medical Education (Chicago: American Medical Association, 1966).

28. Editorial, "The Core Content of Family Medicine, a Report of the Committee on Requirements for Certification," *GP* 34 (1966): 225.

29. John P. Geyman, *Family Practice: Foundation of Changing Health Care*, 2d ed. (Norwalk, Conn.: Appleton-Century-Crofts, 1985).

30. Ibid., 262.

31. Ibid., 263.

32. Ibid., 144.

33. Ibid.

34. Ibid., 262, figure 14–2.

35. Ibid., 241–59.

36. K. M. Fickenscher, "Medical Education and Rural Health Care: Responsibilities and Opportunities," presentation at AAMC Annual Meeting, November 1989 (in press).

37. W. Douglas Skelton, "Primary Care Education and Service: The Role of Medical Schools," speech delivered at the AAMC Council of Deans, Spring Meeting, Sanibel Harbour Resort, Florida, April 1990.

38. H. J. Geiger, "The Neighborhood Health Center: Education of Faculty in Preventive Medicine," *Arch. of Environmental Health* 140 (1967): 912–16.

39. *AAMC Weekly Report* 3, no. 42 (November 30, 1989).

4
Governmental Support for Medical Schools

The dominance of federal research funding for medical schools has been a major determinant of the current status of American medicine, insofar as it has become predominantly specialized and particularly focused on high technology and tertiary care. With federal funding of medical education, as such, now virtually nonexistent, and with research proficiency having the greatest weight in determining recruitment and promotion of faculty, young physicians choosing careers in academic medicine usually start with fellowships in postgraduate training programs supported by NIH research training grants. The majority of medical students, who choose to train for medical specialty practice and are thus less likely to seek research training, compete for the best specialty residency programs to which they can reasonably aspire. These residencies in fields such as internal medicine or surgery, often sponsored by ambitious community hospitals not heavily endowed with NIH funding, emulate the academic medical center's training style and content. Hence, the system is such that virtually every approved specialty residency program is part of a research-based hierarchy stemming from an academic medical center. This has resulted in a situation in which an intelligent patient, walking into a specialist's office and reading the medical school diplomas and residency certificates on the waiting room wall, can be reasonably certain that the care about to be received is up to national standards and is essentially identical to that which would be experienced at the academic medical center itself. Furthermore, specialists belong to national specialty societies or academies through which periodic continuing education courses are provided, and they read relevant journals—all of which tends to assure maintenance of proficiency at a fairly uniform level. With proper selection of a physician and the intelligent scrutiny of credentials, the literate American patient endowed with the financial means for reimbursement for care has an excellent chance of obtaining state-of-the-art diagnosis and treatment.

Clearly, the more restricted the specialty the better this assurance of quality patient care works. With but one organ or system involved, the research is more specific and quantifiable than in the case of general internal medicine, pediatrics, or surgery. In the general specialties which also have primary care as part of their practices, the impact of organ or system-specific research is diluted. Continuing education for generalists requires that individual practitioners seek out those areas in which they feel the need for more training or knowledge. It is, of course, this kind of dilemma that tends to stimulate some generalists, including family physicians, to opt for more specialization within their practices. More variation in performance can therefore be expected at the generalist level than in the highly specialized fields of any of the main branches of medicine.

In any case, in spite of the negative aspects of medicine based almost totally on biomedical science, the degree to which the centrality of research at the academic level has influenced not only medical education but the entire scope of medicine and health throughout the United States and, indeed, the entire world, is one of our great accomplishments.

GERMANY THE SOURCE OF THE RESEARCH CONCEPT

Research has been the faculty activity claiming the highest value ever since the revolution which overtook American colleges of medicine at the end of the nineteenth century. Prior to that time, medical research activity had been essentially limited to the laboratories of a few universities, and there had been little carryover of such research findings to clinical medicine. Even in medical schools attached to universities such as Harvard and Pennsylvania, physicians were trained in physician-controlled settings that were essentially devoid of any effective link to academe. Many of these schools were entirely free-standing, with curriculum and tuition established by the practitioner-faculty who also used and distributed the profits.

Throughout the century, elite and ambitious American physicians had traveled to Scotland, England, France, and Germany either for their basic training as physicians, or for graduate experiences. In the 1890s, partly because of the beginning recognition of the seminal work of such German investigators as Rudolph Virchow and Robert Koch, there was a veritable migration of American physicians to Germany for advanced study. The adoption of research as a major endeavor in American medical schools was strongly stimulated by the return of academically-oriented physicians who had studied in Germany. Many returned filled with enthusiasm for what they had found there; not only high academic standards for medical students but also successful integration of biomedical research into the process of medical education. The numbers of physicians going abroad and their experiences are well described by

Bonner, who estimates the number to have made this pilgrimage during these thirty or so years as upwards of 15,000.[1]

American physicians discovered an academic scene well larded with productive investigators currently discovering a multitude of phenomena both new and relevant to human health.[2] They also discovered a medical profession, largely drawn from the upper classes, enjoying social positions quite different from those typically prevalent at home. Their incomes were higher than what could be expected in the United States, and there were relatively fewer medical schools. The AMA, founded in 1849 with medical education as one of its objectives, had for some time been running articles in the *JAMA* urging a reduction of numbers of American schools.[3] Lower-class physicians were likely to be equated with quacks, and the presence of women and minorities among their ranks was not always productive of joy. Therefore, the notion that research could now be developed as a proper basis for medical education, that this would insure a more difficult preclinical experience, and that many schools would be forced into closing, was a package enthusiastically embraced by most physicians.

Ludmerer has documented the history of medical education reforms at such schools as Harvard, Pennsylvania, and Michigan during the 1870s and 1880s which led to what he refers to as "the most spectacular innovation in the history of American medical education: the opening of the Johns Hopkins Medical School in 1893."[4] This institution was well funded from the start, with a bequest of $7 million from Mr. Johns Hopkins, a Baltimore merchant, banker, and railroad magnate. The new university, led by President Daniel Gilman and founded on the German research-oriented model, recruited outstanding scholars and scientists. The new medical school, whose initial curriculum is said to have been written by Gilman himself, was to be incorporated into the greater university and intended to be the premier school of the nation.

WILLIAM WELCH AND THE JOHNS HOPKINS UNIVERSITY

Among the first and better-known investigators at Hopkins was William Welch, who joined the institution in 1885 after having been to Germany. He returned with an eye to this new medical school as his academic home.[5] He had entered the College of Physicians and Surgeons in New York in 1872, and was appointed prosector to the anatomists in his second year. He graduated in 1875 and began an internship at Bellevue, where he came under the influence of Francis Delafield, a well-known and competent pathologist. In 1876, with substantial help from friends, he sailed for Europe. There he remained until 1885, when he returned in the fall to Baltimore and the Hopkins. The hospital opened its doors in May; Welch remained there until the opening of the medical school in the fall of 1893.

Initially chair of pathology, he helped set the high standards of scholarship and research productivity that applied as the other basic scientists and clinicians were recruited. He spent his entire professional life at the Hopkins, ultimately becoming dean.

The initial Hopkins medical faculty, many of whom had studied in Germany and were exceedingly well trained in their disciplines, felt that education, as they had experienced it in Germany, should be free of rigid structure and be developed according to the needs of students. The educational program developed from the idea that the students themselves were motivated to learn on their own with faculty on hand as advisors and counselors. This new school was founded not only with the idea that it should demonstrate the value of good science as the basis for good medical education, but also that education itself was basically the province of the learner rather than the teacher.[6] It appears that it was from these men that Flexner acquired the medical educational concepts that appear in his report, since it was essentially the Hopkins faculty that he had consulted prior to its authorship. The experience and convictions of the Hopkins medical faculty were probably also the source of his repeated statements about the essential nature of research for quality medical education. The professors themselves had learned their science in this way, so this was the way for their medical students as well.

NEED FOR FUNDING FOR RESEARCH: BEGINNINGS OF A NATIONAL RESOURCE

The National Academy of Science was founded in 1863 as the result of a Civil War emergency. This was an independent but official advisory body authorized to report on any matters relating to the arts and sciences.[7] The first substantial government research funds after the Civil War went to agriculture and were linked to the 1862 Morrill Act. This was followed by research grants to state agricultural experiment stations. Indeed, some of the first contributions made by federal scientists to medicine came from the Department of Agriculture. An example was the work of Theobald Smith who, in 1889, demonstrated the relationship between Texas Fever and tick bites.

A National Board of Health was established in 1879 and supported investigation on such diseases as yellow fever. It had no political influence, was opposed by the Marine Hospital Service, and was abolished after three years. It did hold a 1882 conference on uniform disease nomenclature (nosology), a subject that had been urged by the AMA. In cooperation with the Royal College of Surgeons, it revised the system and published the International List of Causes of Death.

In 1887 a bacteriology laboratory, known as the Laboratory of Hygiene, was established under Dr. Joseph J. Kinyoun at the Marine Hospital on Staten Island for research on cholera and other infectious diseases. It was redesignated the Hygienic Laboratory in 1891, and much later was moved to Bethesda, Maryland, where it was renamed the National Institute of Health.

An Army Medical School had been started in the mid-1890s as a research and teaching center. At the close of the Civil War, John S. Billings, later to have a major position in the Johns Hopkins Hospital, had been put in charge of the Surgeon General's Library, where he built up a fine collection, and in 1887 introduced the Index Medicus. The Census Bureau was set up in 1902, and birth registrations began in 1915.

In 1908 the Hospital Service had become the United States Public Health Service, and in 1912 the service's research interests were encouraged by Congress which authorized it to "study and investigate the diseases of man and conditions influencing the propagation and spread thereof." Valuable studies were thereafter made on malaria, hookworm, trachoma, and plague. Notable among individual investigations were those of Edward Francis on tularemia and Joseph Goldberger on pellagra.

In 1930, the importance of the service's research program was recognized by Congress through the Ransdell Act, which stipulated that the Hygiene Laboratory move to Bethesda, and that it fuse with the National Institute of Health.[8] The act also authorized $750,000 for the construction of two NIH buildings, and created a system of fellowships. The future of this institution as a national research center thus seemed assured.

THE PRIVATE SECTOR AND FOUNDATIONS

At that time the private sector was active as well. Pharmaceutical houses were among the leaders in the support of medical research and by 1880 had amassed a great deal of money. There were essentially two kinds of corporations. There were those such as Abbott and Parke Davis whose products were largely distributed by physicians' prescription, and there was also a group of patent medicine concerns whose products flooded the country. Shryock estimates that by 1880 these companies had amassed capital of over $28 million and an annual value of products of more than $38 million. No accounting is available of how this money was distributed.

Foundations became the first and most effective outside support system for medical schools in their early years. Schools now being planned were not only complicated in terms of diversity of personnel but were also very expensive, particularly in faculty, staff, space, and equipment for the preclinical phase of medical education, where a whole new array of disciplines needed to be discovered and taught. While required funding was not usually available from normal sources, the foundations could be invoked to provide seed money for new schools and catalytic dollars for those schools attempting to reform according to the new standards.

Leading this interest in health profession education was the Rockefeller Foundation which, even after three years' effort, had failed to obtain a federal charter, and so had become incorporated in the State of New York in 1913. Beginning with about $3 million, it possessed roughly $182 million in 1927 and, by 1940, had dispensed a grand total of over $323 million. It became interested in public health as well, attacked the Southern hookworm problem, and in 1916 founded The Johns Hopkins School of Hygiene and Public Health. This was the first research-based school of public health in the United States.

Other foundations supporting medical education in particular and health in general included the Commonwealth Fund, the Carnegie Foundation, and the Markle Foundation. While an exact accounting of the total amount granted to medical schools and universities is not readily available, it seems clear that the main effort of the foundations was expended on a few private schools in the East and Midwest, and that that the level of support was inadequate for any sort of broadly-based sustained research effort.

ACADEMIC MEDICINE AS A CAREER

The financial status of medical school faculty lacking independent financial means during these early days of reform in medical education is somewhat obscure. It is certain that the level of financial support available from universities and private sources was low, and it seems probable that some form of consultation practice for academic clinicians was permitted. For basic scientists without such an available income source, subsisting on academic salaries alone must have been difficult. It is my impression that the pure academic life was most comfortably suited to those with independent means, and that this situation continued until after the second World War.

Nonetheless, especially in the relatively wealthy private schools in the East where research was largely funded by foundations, other philanthropy, or outright gifts from industry, there was great research progress. Discoveries included immunization against diphtheria, insulin for diabetes, pneumococcal typing and type-specific serum for treatment of pneumonia, diagnostic and therapeutic radiology, and considerable advancement of anesthesiological and surgical knowledge, equipment, and techniques. The present situation in which medical research is concentrated on projects related to fundamental processes often most relevant to rare diseases had not yet come to pass. Academic research between the two world wars was focusing on the major concerns of both the public and the practicing medical profession. Thus, while times were difficult from the standpoint of research funding, the later-developing dissonance between the preclinical and clinical years was not yet in evidence, and medical education proceeded without serious crises.

My own recollections of the status of research in medical schools and teaching hospitals go back to the late 1930s when, as a medical student, I spent two summers working at the University of Pennsylvania with radiologists who were collaborating with anatomists and orthopedists in the study of certain features of radiologic imaging of the spine. While funds were apparently provided by the medical school for equipment and technicians in the anatomy department, there was no such research laboratory in radiology. Furnishings were sparse, and much of what we did was with improvised ad hoc procedures and homemade gear. Later, in the mid-1940s as chief resident at the Children's Hospital of Philadelphia and a young faculty member, it was incumbent on me to become involved in a research project. This was before the ever-present availability of the NIH as a funding source had emerged, and our grant for the clinical pharmacology of antibiotics in children was obtained from the Army's Division of Chemical Warfare, based in Fort Dietrick, Maryland. (Their interest in such investigation related to its possible usefulness in the event of a gas attack on the United States.) Later, as the panoply of antibiotics expanded from penicillin and streptomycin to such drugs as aureomycin and chloramphenicol, our project was supported by relevant drug companies who, incidentally, became disenchanted with us when our data did not support their claims of efficacy with much smaller doses than those we were recommending. The procedures for obtaining government grants, including formal application, peer review, and competitive awards, were still several years away.

ROOSEVELT, SCIENCE, AND THE FEDERAL GOVERNMENT

Franklin Roosevelt had been elected president in 1934, and had appointed a Science Advisory Board of more than one hundred scientists and engineers to survey the general relations of government and research. This was the first attempt to assay the complex research situation on a national scale. Its 1935 report was in many ways critical. It concluded, however, that no comprehensive, centrally controlled research program was desirable in this country. It held that certain problems (such as those in public health) required national action, while in other fields federal studies could supplement those of private institutions. It warned against political interference in research, and recommended the appointment of a permanent nonpolitical advisory board to work with the various agencies and to advise the Bureau of the Budget in relation to research appropriations.

The next step was taken in 1937 with the reorganization of the

NIH into a number of divisions, and with the passage of the National Cancer Institute Act, signed by President Roosevelt on August 5.[9] The cornerstone for Building 1 on the Bethesda campus was laid in 1938, Mr. and Mrs. Luke Wilson began a series of grants in the form of land, and Congress approved construction of new, larger laboratory facilities. The institute took on functions somewhat similar to those of medical schools and foundations, and it provided technical training for specialists, offered fellowships within the service, and distributed grants-in-aid. In order to keep in touch with and stimulate research, the institute considered 137 applications for grants between 1938 and 1940, and awarded 33 grants with a total of $220,000.

On the eve of World War II, the National Academy of Science numbered about 220 members representing 95 constituent societies; more than 1100 other members served on its various committees. From this group of scientists a number of effective and prestigious committees were formed, such as the National Defense Research Committee. To coordinate the medical sciences, an analogous committee—the Committee on Medical Research—was appointed. By the end of 1944 it had become responsible for the distribution of over $15 million. Never before, except possibly in Russia, had such sums been made available for medical research. Contracts were made with investigators in institutes and universities, and were administered with funds delegated to the executive secretary of the Office of Scientific Research.

The war accelerated the testing and application of knowledge derived from peacetime studies and included such advances as better methods of destroying bacteria in the air of military quarters, new and potent bubonic plague vaccine, cholera vaccine, sulfonamide treatment of dysentery, gas gangrene toxoids, anti-streptococcal sera, better influenza vaccine, and penicillin for the treatment of syphilis. Indeed, the most striking achievement of the whole program may have been the development of this antibiotic. While the discovery and early work on this substance was performed in Britain, its massive production was an American feat. The Army death rate from disease declined from the 1917 figure of 14.1 percent to 0.06 percent; 97 percent of wounded men survived.

Just prior to 1940, the total research expenditures in the country had been about $250 million, of which but $50 million had been federal funds; by 1944 more than $600 million was being spent by the federal government alone. Senator Kilgore, as chair of the relevant subcommittee, summarized it all, and noted a lack of coordination of federal programs.[10] The survey's main purpose was to develop a legislative base for research funding. Research momentum should not be lost, as had occurred in 1919. The report recommended legislation with respect to (1) better coordination of research for national defense, (2) maximum use of federal wartime research for peacetime production, and (3) maintenance of research activity in economic fields of particular national concern. A program for this legislation was later introduced by the subcommittee, which emphasized the essential nature of both basic and applied studies. There was also considerable concern about matters inherent in government control such as the hazards of regimentation of science.

Roosevelt, sympathetic to both science and social planning, wrote to Vannevar Bush, director of the Office of Scientific Research, commenting on his organization's unique experience in coordinating war research and inquired why the lessons so acquired could not also be applied in peacetime. He requested a recommendation for federal measures that would (1) make research useful to the public as soon as possible, and (2) enable the federal government best to aid research in public and private institutions. He added: "With particular reference to the war of science against disease, what can be done now to organize a program for continuing in the future the work which has been done in medicine and related sciences?"[11]

THE NATIONAL SCIENCE FOUNDATION

The response from Bush was a publication entitled *Science, the Endless Frontier.*[12] This turned out to be the origin of the National Science Foundation. The text was a statement on why such a federal agency was needed. It indicated that, while the responsibility for research lay fundamentally with the medical schools and universities, their shrunken budgets and programs left little remaining to carry out this important mission. Endowment income, foundation grants, and private donations were all diminishing with no immediate prospect of a change in this trend while the cost of medical research had risen. The government should extend financial support for basic medical research to these institutions. A new agency was needed to cope with this task.

Medical schools and universities, furthermore, had an obligation to provide the individual worker with the opportunity for free, untrammeled study of nature,

in the directions and by the methods suggested by his interests, curiosity, and imagination.... It is the special province of the medical schools and universities to foster medical research in this way ... a duty which cannot be shifted to Government agencies, industrial organizations, or to any other institutions."[13]

This call for research involvement was not limited to the elite institutions, but included the entire spectrum of medical schools. Indeed, he commented that most of the work hitherto had been done by the large schools, and that "this should be corrected by building up the weaker institutions, especially in regions which now have no strong medical research activities."[14]

In other words, all medical schools needed to develop their research possibilities with the help of the federal establishment. Again, after the calamitous impact of World War II, the idea was reiterated that every school and university, regardless of its location or self-stated and developed goals, should be a repository of important medical research, regardless of impact on its institutional educational programs. The idea that research and teaching are entirely compatible efforts was again strongly affirmed.

While Bush's document was a major prelude to the subsequent explosion in the government's research support of medical schools, the political process would later focus NSF activity on funding basic research in university science departments and research institutes. The NIH was on the verge of its enormous growth toward preeminence in extramural funding and intramural conduct of medical research.

1946: TRANSFER OF WARTIME FUNDS TO NIH

As the war drew to a close, discussion about the ultimate recipients of the grants and contracts was managed through the Committee on Medical Research chaired by A. N. Richards, a famous University of Pennsylvania physiologist. In January 1946 the committee met for a final series of important meetings. Although it did not expire until the following year, its wartime mission was accomplished.[15] Dr. Richards had presided over the dispensation of $25 million during the life of the committee. Now, he met with but three government representatives; one each from the Navy, the Army, and the PHS on behalf of the NIH. The process was such that the NIH ended up the recipient of almost all of the money.

The significance of the transfer is most easily seen in dollar terms. From an expenditure of $180,000 for research projects in fiscal 1945, the figure went to $850,000 for fiscal 1946 and in 1947, the year most of the contracts were transferred, to $4,000,000. With its new statutory authority, and its new contracts, the agency needed more manpower and a bigger administrative budget. In the same year, calendar 1946, the Congress appropriated for NIH for fiscal 1947 almost $8,000,000— more than a tenfold increase since the start of the War and almost four times what its budget had been when the Japanese surrendered to General MacArthur in August 1945.[16]

THE NEW LAY CONSTITUENCY

As the structure for a major governmental support system for research in America's medical schools came into being, a significant lay constituency for such a development also emerged. In 1942, Mrs. Albert D. Lasker (Mary) formed a foundation devoted to increasing the funding of research in medicine, particularly cancer. She persuaded her husband to join her in establishing such a foundation, and put up $50,000. The foundation "shortly commenced an annual series of awards to medical and biological scientists whose research efforts advanced the cause of better health, awards that became as prestigious as any given in the U.S."

In 1945, Mary Lasker and others began fund-raising campaigns for the American Society for the Control of Cancer (which later became the American Cancer Society) for which they raised $10 million in 1946. This accomplishment led to generating Mrs. Lasker's two firmly held convictions: namely, that the American public would support a major research effort to a far greater degree than had ever been realized, and that even greatly increased amounts of private money would be inadequate to make maximum headway against most of the nation's disease, so that the federal government must become a major continuing participant in the cause.[17]

Strickland states, for example:

> Because ours has been a research-conscious, even research-oriented society since World War II, it is easy to forget that before Pearl Harbor research was not in a position of high visibility or universally accepted value in our country. In the universities, soon to house laboratories often involving large teams of scientists, research before the War was but a fractional part of normal campus activity. It was an activity usually small and personal, often disjointed and sometimes, by some academicians, disdained.[18]

During this era, then, there was great pressure placed on Congress through hearings, personal involvement, and in whatever fashion a lay group such as this could be effective. Mrs. Margaret Mahoney became involved, and the time when this

> Lasker-Mahoney combine began its operations in 1944, was one in which most laboratory researchers and their sponsors were satisfied with the current pace of progress. Those directing wartime research activities were divided on the need for continuing large-scale, special federal programs; private agencies were concentrating on care and prevention, but not on cure through research; and members of Congress evidenced only occasional concern, generally coinciding with periodic outbursts of popular enthusiasm, and were ambivalent if not confused in the face of various research policy approaches being advanced.[19]

It seems, then, that in some ways the informed lay public was ahead of both Congress and at least some scientists, and that the Lasker-congressional faction was of great importance in getting much of today's funding apparatus into place.

GENERAL MEDICAL CARE LEGISLATION

Meanwhile, during the Truman administration, a congressional drive developed for a medical care bill. A congressional leadership structure had formed, and there seemed little reason to suspect that the bill generated with their support would fail, since it seemed designed to insure universal access to medical care. Even with the predictable AMA opposition, the possibility for success seemed good for this legislation, the Wagner-Murray-Dingell bill. A major reason for its demise appears to have been its encumbrance with specific items of aid to medical education, which the AMA adamantly opposed. Continued AMA opposition, together with the advent of the Korean War in 1950, led to its ultimate defeat. With the federal government safely out of the funding mechanisms for medical care and education, the way was cleared for the AMA to remain essentially neutral on the issue of increased federal funding of research. The AMA, then, would remain politically uninvolved in the great national research enterprise which has done so much to advance health and the practice of medicine.

The original thinking by Flexner, the founding Hopkins faculty, and others on behalf of the elevation of research to a central position in medical educational activity included the concept that research problem-solving methodology was virtually identical to that of problem solving in clinical medicine. Mastery of the logic inherent in research, then, was essential not only for learning but also for practicing scientific medicine. It is at least ironic, if not tragic, that a governmental plan encompassing the unity of medical care, research, and education was converted, largely through the influence of organized medicine, into three separate political compartments. The notion that part of this trichotomy could be resolved to the benefit of medical schools by extending the scope of research grants to educational or other relevant purposes, while successful for a time, was soon halted when interested congressional committees discovered the ploy.

The political process, free of obligation to become seriously involved in financing medical care or education, was then able to concentrate on the relatively uncontroversial task of developing a national edifice and support mechanism for biomedical research. Except for the advent of the categorical Medicare and Medicaid programs in the 1960s, this trend has continued to the present. We continue, furthermore, to pay an escalating price for this disjointed social inadequacy in costly and depressing health and medical care inequities, with little evidence of a comprehensive solution in sight.

THE NIH AS THE MAJOR SOURCE OF MEDICALLY-RELATED RESEARCH FUNDING

Not until several years after the war were the precise sources of federal funds for university and medical school research really identified. In 1950 Truman signed the law creating the National Science Foundation within which was a Division of Biological and Medical Sciences. In the same year, Congress passed the Omnibus Medical

Research Act, which not only authorized the establishment of the Institute of Arthritis and Metabolic Diseases but gave the surgeon general authority to establish additional institutes. It was finally resolved that the mission of the NIH and its institutes would be disease-oriented and supportive of relevant basic and applied research. The National Science Foundation would concentrate on basic research for the purpose of advancing knowledge and understanding of science not necessarily related to medicine.

The NIH, then, was not to be the sole agent for support of medical research. The NSF was to have some role, and the Atomic Energy Commission was directed by Congress to look into the possibility of relating atomic research to cancer cure. The Veterans' Administration and the Defense Department had also become involved. Several federal agencies were thus to be in support of research, with any future aid for education to come from an as yet unidentified source. The NIH, nonetheless, would ultimately become the main reservoir of funds for health-related research programs.

Lyndon Johnson had been vice-president during the Kennedy administration and, after his election, espoused many causes that had been Kennedy's. In general, his goals for the "Great Society" included elimination of poverty, provision of greater educational and employment opportunities for the needy, and improvement of education, research, and medical care. Among his main efforts was the passage of a series of laws that dealt with such issues as a national health planning program, utilization of medical schools as regional health centers, and the promotion of medical research from sources other than those normally the province of the NIH. During this brief time before the Vietnam War had escalated to an unmanageable degree, a flood of legislation appeared. While none was clearly earmarked for the process of medical education, some was leaning in that direction. Funds which could easily be manipulated into educational ventures became available for educational research, distributed academic health centers, and various other such programs. Of particular interest to many deans was the package oriented around curriculum modification that was linked to enrollment expansion.[20] This was an exciting though anxious time, fraught with tumult from protests about the Vietnam War, the growing intensity of the Cold War, the proper role for the American military machine, and the near certainty that the Great Society would ultimately collapse unless the war was soon settled. For many of us in new medical schools, the programs fit well with our own efforts, though we were constantly aware of the likelihood of our ultimate entrapment in the fiscal morass borne of attempting simultaneous public support of brave social programs and vast military operations. This period was nonetheless the high point of federal contribution to medical care programs linked to medical education. The likelihood of such a time recurring in the foreseeable future seems remote indeed.

The growth of the NIH, on the other hand, has proceeded apace under some extraordinarily good leadership. James Shannon held the position of director from 1955 until 1968. He was followed by Robert Marston, who was in charge until 1973; Robert Stone, who remained until 1975; Donald Fredrickson, from 1975 until 1981; and James Wyngaarden, who was director from 1981 until 1989. Current NIH funding is over $7 billion.[21]

The National Library of Medicine became a component of NIH in 1968. Its past history stemmed from 1836 when the Library of the Office of the Surgeon General was established. In 1922 it had become the Army Medical Library, and in 1952 the Armed Forces Medical Library. In 1956 it became the National Library of Medicine and was placed under the Public Health Service. The new building in Bethesda was dedicated in 1961 and, thereafter, it has become integrated with most medical school and science libraries in the United States.

The Warren Grant Magnuson Clinical Center, whose construction was started in 1948, is the organization's hospital and center for clinical research. It has 540 beds, and facilities and support services for nearly 1,200 physicians working for all of the NIH institutes with intramural research programs. Its proximity to research laboratories provides quick transfer of laboratory information and ideas to the patient and is, indeed, the site of much productive investigation. In addition to research and patient care, the center offers opportunities for advanced training for young physicians and other health care students. Patients related to virtually all institutes are admitted, and the results of various projects are published in regular medical journals. Patients are generally admitted free of charge, and one gets the impression that the quality of care is of the highest order.[22] It is in this center that some of the most significant investigation in medicine has occurred.

THE INITIATIVES OF THE JOHNSON ADMINISTRATION

Lingering doubts among some congressmen about the compatibility of research and medical teaching could have been resolved had, for example, the Wagner-Murray-Dingell bill passed in 1950. In that case, funds for education would have been regularly included in budget authorizations within the scope and intent of the legislation. With Johnson in the White House, however, a new surge of socially-oriented energy was in the air. Part of this energy was directed toward improvement of the nation's health and medical care, with the aged and the poor at the forefront of the effort. The AMA was on the verge of a significant political defeat, since it had vigorously and publicly opposed the passage of Medicare legislation. This program became law in 1965; Medicaid, a companion program to provide medical care to certain categories of the poor, was passed shortly thereafter. Robert Kennedy, as attorney general, was developing health programs for the poor emanating from his Office of Economic Opportunity.

With the certainty of an increased need for physicians now apparent, the issue of federal help for medical schools became more urgent. In August 1968 a significant breakthrough came with the passage of P.L. 90–490, which achieved the endorsement of both the AAMC and the AMA. Having been convinced of the reality of the serious physician shortage and of the need for more educational emphasis on primary care, the AMA had by then relinquished some of its antipathy toward federal aid to medical education. Construction funding was authorized in the amount of $170 million for fiscal 1970 and $225 million for 1971. Two-to-one matching between federal and state funds was now required. There were special features such as "institutional grants" to replace the previous "basic improvement grants"; each school was granted $25,000, and all schools shared in a distribution of $550 per student.[23] An annual series of similar public laws followed, finally fading out in 1977 and disappearing altogether in 1980.[24] No federal support of this nature has since been forthcoming. These funds were exceedingly useful to deans and faculty of new medical schools, and those where innovations in teaching were being attempted.

BACK TO FEDERAL CONSERVATISM: A PAUSE IN EDUCATIONAL FUNDING, AND CONTINUED INCREASE IN DOLLARS FOR RESEARCH

Following Johnson came a conservative swing with the election of Richard Nixon to the presidency. Subtle changes occurred, such as the affirmative action emphasis on gender in addition to race, federal endorsement of Health Maintenance Organizations (HMOs), and the beginning of newly found enthusiasm for private enterprise and competition in the field of medical care. Institutional grants focused on educational improvement and program development essentially disappeared; the mainstay of the government's support system for medical education generally reverted to research alone.

Since the beginning of the Nixon administration to the present, the NIH's obligations from appropriations have increased from $2 billion to over $7 billion. In addition, there has been a concomitant development of other sources of research funding for medical schools, such as the Hughes Foundation, and various contributions from other governmental sources.

The impact of this greatly expanded source of research funding on the medical schools was significant. Lippard, for example, wrote:

The average faculty member had to adapt to a new way of life. Instead of working in the laboratory as an individual, he became the manager of a research team consisting of more junior faculty members, postdoctoral fellows, technicians, and secretaries. Skill in composing research proposals often determined his recognition and advancement. He was on a treadmill, constantly concerned over his current grant, and over the preparation of an equally inspired application for renewal when it expired. His loyalty to the school tended to diminish as he became dependent on outside sources for support of his research, and often for at least a portion of his salary. If local conditions were not to his liking he could pack up and move to another institution, taking his support and auxiliary personnel with him.[25]

Faculty thus tended to become more dependent on the willingness of the NIH to provide funds in the forms of grants than on the parent institution itself for support.

The conflict between the perceived drudgery of teaching and the intellectual satisfaction of research, as evident in the late 1950s, is revealed by Miller, who wrote:

Another area of personal conflict and insecurity is the teaching-research incongruity. In the undergraduate college the teacher is hired to teach but receives professional rewards for publishing the results of his research. In medical schools it sometimes seems that teaching is regarded as a byproduct of research and not a major independent responsibility. Under such a circumstance, it is not unexpected to find that faculty members exhibit some reluctance to giving time to students, to course preparation, to committee assignments, since these activities do not add to their stature. . . . The term productivity in academic circles has almost become synonymous with research productivity.[26]

This should be read in contrast to the picture of the satisfaction with the lifestyle of pure research within the intramural program of the NIH. For example:

The very compactness of the Bethesda campus and the willingness of its immunologists to work together, to have seminars constantly, and wander in and out of each others' labs gave them a leg up. At centers where in-house competition was fiercer, such as Harvard, people were more secretive. At the state universities the sheer number of researchers, however excellent they were individually, did not achieve that critical mass.[27]

Such a statement, of course, brings up the crucial question of whether the university is always the ideal location for major basic research.

Today the NIH is staffed by some 12,000 employees, including more than 3,200 scientists. Its budget, which exceeds $7 billion, supports far more than the buildings, laboratories, and people on the Bethesda campus. More than 80 % of the NIH annual budget funds the work of nearly 50,000 scientists in 1650 universities, medical schools, hospitals, and other research institutions throughout the United States and abroad.[28]

This statement was included in a commemoration of the NIH's one hundredth anniversary. Although the institutes are vulnerable to some criticism in their categorization by disease, age, or organ, the skillful coordination of their intramural and extramural programs, and the degree to which peer review and fairness in the competitive grant awarding process have set worldwide examples. There is no question that the nation's preeminence in science and medicine is to an extraordinary degree dependent on this national accomplishment.

CONTROL OF NIH GRANTS BY MEDICAL FACULTIES

Wyngaarden lauds the 3,200 scientists in Bethesda and the 50,000 who have received institute grants. It is true, however, that many of these scientists function as part of the institutes' support system as members of study sections and other committees relevant to grant priorities, peer review of grant applications, and the actual awarding of grants. Institute directors are usually drawn from this population, and the scientific rules and guidelines generally reflect the standards and values of academe.

Is this research support mechanism, then, totally controlled and operated by the scientific population whom it supports? Probably not, since Congress controls the purse and sits in judgment of the NIH's performance. During the late 1950s and early 1960s, for example, a congressional committee became active vis-à-vis the administration of grants in medical schools and other research institutions. Its members felt that some money was being spent unwisely, i.e., was being siphoned off for educational purposes. New rules were established and such diversion of funds has diminished. By and large, though, Congress has been friendly to the institutes and, as long as the public retains its faith in and enthusiasm for medical research, their future seems filled with promise.

CONFLICT BETWEEN EDUCATION AND RESEARCH
CONTINUES

While the research support accruing to medical schools through the NIH seems secure (with dips and variations depending on fluctuations in available funds), we are still left with the problem of conflict with the basic educational purposes of medical school faculties. The assumption had been made, accepted, and often reiterated that research and teaching are entirely compatible and that there is basically no conflict. This had been asserted by such important persons as William Welch, Abraham Flexner and, more recently, by Vannevar Bush. It also seems entirely probable that such had been accepted by the members of Congress voting for the NIH appropriations. This idea of research-teaching compatibility remains an article of faith with many faculty members today.

Indeed, the impact of the NIH on medical school faculties has been great. For example, Ludmerer states:

> The first and second generation medical educators envisioned a university spirit pervading all of a school's activities, but they saw research, teaching, and patient care as closely and harmoniously intertwined. Little did they foresee the degree to which research would come to dominate the American medical school or how semi-autonomous research institutes would be created within the schools.[29]

The degree to which research has dominated the American medical school is also described by Rothstein, who states that fulltime basic science faculty increased from 1,656 in 1951 to 13,783 in 1984, and that clinical fulltime faculty increased from 2,277 to 44,984 during the same period.[30] He feels that the larger growth in clinical faculty is more a function of increased volume of clinical practice than of research intensity. The growth in basic science faculty, however, is probably mostly attributable to increased research funding. He points out that this degree of growth significantly outstrips the number of medical, allied health, nursing, and other kinds of students for whom they have been teachers. For example: "Using other data, between 1963–64 and 1970–71, the number of full time equivalent (FTE) faculty increased by 83.2 percent, from 14,468 to 26,504, while the number of FTE students of all kinds increased by only 40.2 percent, from 69,929 to 98,012."

A quantitative statement on the impact of research funding on medical education was obtained from the AAMC Washington office.[31] In order of rank, the schools range in dollars spent on research in 1985–86 from $112 million, to a low of less than $1 million. With the number of schools at 127, the median institution had a research budget of $12 million during 1985–86. In terms of growth, the following indicates the dimension of this phenomenon. The school in the number one position ($112 million) grew from $24 million in 1972–73 to its present status—roughly fivefold. The school in the median position grew from $2.8 million to its present level of $12 million—also about fivefold. Indeed, comparable growth rates in NIH research funding extend to virtually all medical schools.

The Association of Professors of Medicine (APM) and the AAMC have recently completed a study on the research activity of fulltime faculty in departments of medicine.[32] All such departments in the United States were surveyed, with a high level of completed responses. Although only 20 percent of all internal medicine faculty spend at least 50 percent of their time in research, approximately 50 percent of the faculty are, in fact, engaged in research activities that account for at least 20 percent of their time. The conclusion

94

that "the modern department of medicine is geared for major roles in patient care and teaching"[33] may be true, but the study, it seems to me, needs to be extended with more precise attention paid to these other two activities. The questionnaire completed by each faculty member contained an item—"Major Areas of Responsibility"[34]—which listed other activities, i.e., instruction, research, patient care (patient education), administration, and other professional activities. While neat, and apparently covering all bases, it fails to explore some relevant variables—for example, the time and energy consumed in the planning of and participation in a seminar or group process sequence compared with that needed to give a lecture course. Likewise, if the curriculum is really oriented around student needs, a multitude of meetings and special preparation may be needed. The time and energy devoted to patient care is likewise left unquantified and needs further elaboration. Thus, while the study's printed conclusion as to its implications may turn out to be correct, such conclusions may have been drawn prematurely.

In 1960 the Carnegie Commission on Higher Education and the Nation's Health published a short report on academic medical centers as locations for health professional education, and recommended the formation of over one hundred new centers. The report affirms its support of expanding medical education through more health centers, but with the following reservations:

> The Commission believes that a vigorous biomedical research program is essential for continued progress in combating disease and that it is an integral component of the process of medical and dental education. Our recommendations above for cost-of-instruction supplements to support this educational process are predicated on the continuation of federal support for biomedical research and for studies of the needed changes in health manpower education and the delivery of health care.[35]

It is the view of the Commission that the total amount provided to university health science centers for research by the Federal Government should be maintained at its current percentage of the GNP (0.042%). Changes in appropriations to reflect changes in the Gross National Product (GNP) should be made on the basis of a moving average of the total GNP in order to avoid abrupt or irregular shifts in amounts. Federal allocations for research should cover the full costs of research projects, since present requirements for institutional contributions frequently result in a diversion of funds from instructional and other expenses. The Commission recommends that not less than 10 percent and not more than 25 percent of the research grants to any university health science center take the form of institutional grants rather than grants for specific research projects.[36]

The report also recommended that funds be made available to

support research on methods of achieving greater efficiency in health manpower education and in the delivery of health care, as well as for biomedical research.

The commission also recommended $2,000 cost of instruction supplements to university health science centers for each medical and dental student enrolled, bonuses for expansion of enrollment, cost-of-instruction supplements to university health science centers and their affiliated hospitals for each house officer, and bonuses for curriculum reform.[37] Here, again, attention was being paid to the cost of instruction which had been seriously affected by inadequate granting practices and university-based accounting procedures.

The Carnegie group met again in 1976 and published a second updated report.[38] Since 1970, for example, the shortage of 50,000 physicians had essentially been eliminated. The total number of active allopathic and osteopathic physicians had risen from about 323,000 to an estimated 378,000. The 1971 Health Manpower legislation was reviewed (P.L. 92–157) with emphasis on the capitation payments of $2500 for each fulltime first-, second-, and third-year student, plus $4000 for each graduate of a four-year curriculum or $6,000 from a three-year program. Such capitation payments were, however, conditional on an increase in first-year students of 10 percent over the enrollment in the fall of 1970. In other words, the costs of education were partially paid, with enrollment increase a condition for such payment. There were also special scholarship awards for students as well as student loans. The report also points out that "research funds, which represent a large proportion of federal aid to university health science centers, are provided under separate legislation, particularly in the form of funds for the National Institutes of Health" (p. 19). Another recommendation was for extending the provisions of existing health-manpower legislation for one year, in order to avoid a disruption of the flow of federal support funds to university health science centers.

This report also discussed costs of medical education using data acquired by the Institute of Medicine, and suggested that funding in the amount of one-third of the educational fraction of tuition should be the federal government's responsibility. This was largely because of the national impact of medical schools, their unequal distribution around the country, and their value as a national resource.

The main impact of this report was similar to that of 1970. It insisted on separation of sources of funding for education and research in order to insure that the maintenance of research programs did not jeopardize education.

John Cooper, influential as always as president of the AAMC, wrote in 1977:

> [Academic medical centers] are also heavily involved with basic and applied research. With their affiliated hospital, they provide a sub-

stantial part of the nation's medical services, most of it tertiary care, and the avenue for introducing advances in the biomedical sciences into clinical medicine. . . .

Faculty members' commitment to the institution qua institution, more badly needed than ever under these circumstances, has been weakened as a consequence of the grant and contract support they obtain individually for their research activities and the magnitude of the income they generate from reimbursements for medical services they render.[39]

Cooper's feelings about the impact of the dollar earned for care of patients is likewise important. Indeed, the numerical dominance of specialists among fulltime faculty, and their skill with the most recent technology, are such as to bring much tertiary-care practice to academic medical centers. Furthermore, it has become fairly routine during recent years for deans to ask their faculties to see more patients in order to cope with the increased costs of medical education and the increased salaries being drawn by these very faculty members. The priorities for education, therefore, have dropped to third on a list of three. Research, with its source extramurally based is presently number one. It is here that the basic sciences turn for their sustenance. Clinicians, on the other hand, while often well endowed with research projects, can turn to patient care for intellectual satisfaction, and the additional income is a major attraction, both to the department and to themselves. Medical student education, especially in the absence of any significant extramural funding in its behalf, is clearly at the bottom of the list.

BASIC SCIENCE DEPARTMENTS

Basic science departments are generally considerably larger than necessary for teaching and faculty responsibilities not related to research. A department chairperson, starting from the beginning in the building process, generates his recruitment and development goals on the basis of national standards of excellence. During his faculty experience he has firmly acquired the concept of the "critical mass" for his discipline. For example, a proper physiology department must feature a considerable portion of the spectrum of physiology's accepted subdivisions. These might include heart, lung, gastrointestinal tract, kidney, and brain, as well as some phase of molecular biology. Including graduate students, fellows, and research assistants, a departmental complement can be large indeed. Since all physiologists are trained in basic physiology, and have shown proficiency in their attainment of doctoral degrees, a teacher from any one of the various subgroups can convey what most medical students need to know. The size and complexity of the department, therefore, generally far exceeds institutional educational needs.

It is in the interest of the institution, however, to support research and the training of graduate students for their own sakes, and budgeting from the dean's office should reflect such goals, with periodic negotiations for allocations of faculty time and effort being an integral part of the management task. In any case, it is unfortunate that total departmental expenditures are sometimes allocated to the cost of teaching students. Advancing medical science is surely a vital part of the social responsibility of medical centers as well as a path to academic distinction.

I feel it is important for budgetary specificity to be applied today, especially in view of the trend toward such new educational initiatives as problem-based learning, in which specific faculty expertise in supervising student-based acquisition of knowledge and problem solving is no longer critical.[40] The apparent impingement of such "soft" use of valuable faculty time may well be interpreted as adversely affecting the "credit hour per fulltime student" calculation on which justification for departmental funding, especially in state institutions, is so often based.

Research, then, is the intellectual life-blood of the basic sciences, and must continue to be supported to the extent that funds, whether intramural or extramural, can be obtained for that purpose. Indeed, it is essential that extensive public support for biomedical research be maintained. Except to the extent that medical students are involved in actual research, the research budget should not be included as part of the cost of medical education. While the tension caused by the competing obligations of teaching and research is probably inevitable, it can be minimized through effective management practices.

At the time President Reagan presented his 1989 budget, the *New York Times* took notice of its inclusion of $10 billion for basic research.[41] While the relevant article failed to clarify how much of this was allocated to the NIH, it revealed the growth of research expenditures from $4.7 billion in 1980 to the present $10 billion. The article showed the president in a white coat "showing his interest in science" and further stated:

> Mr. Reagan sees science as an engine of economic growth, and he seems to have a healthy mystical respect for its potential. He wants to increase support for scientific research even as he seeks to cut spending for housing, community development, mass transit and other social and domestic programs.

Two years of the Bush administration seems to presage continuation of the Reagan domestic priorities. While continued support of research seems secure, there appears little likelihood of new expenditures for medical education, and continuation of the present asymmetrical nature of federal support for academic medicine is predictable.

SUMMARY AND CONCLUSIONS

We are now at the end of the ninth year of conservative presidential leadership. The current status of planning for the 1991 Department of Health and Human Services (HHS) appears not to include the increases in Medicaid funding for which the president campaigned one year ago,[42] and that are urgently needed in such areas as effective attention to the problem of infant mortality. At the same time, the NIH appropriation has been announced at the level of $7.683 billion;[43] a modest but definite increase over the preceding year. It seems clear that research remains the one stable portion of federal funding.

In view of the nation's consistently conservative domestic political preference, it would appear that federal incentives will continue to be directed toward the maintenance of the status quo in the balance between research and education. While it is possible that there will be federal incentives for schools to undertake programs in such arenas as primary care, rural medicine, and extensive research in health care, any major help from government in the foreseeable future seems unlikely. Some help could be expected from foundations, but such support is generally highly specific for selected talented institutions, unless it is awarded to an umbrella organization such as the AAMC. In any case, it cannot be expected that desired change will be attempted in response to federal incentives. The schools themselves, with appropriate help from the AAMC, AMA, and other medically related groups, must develop their own momentum.

We have noted the effectiveness of research not only as the source of most of our new knowledge and technology, but also as the driving force in maintaining coordination, disciplinary cohesion, and a near-guarantee to the public of a standard level of excellence in specialty medicine throughout the nation. Where illness is the result of physical injury, is specific to an organ, system, or body fluid, or where precise, finely tuned use of laboratory and technical skills are major tools for successful diagnosis and treatment, the system is superb.

Research and its fruits are the source of much of the system's excellence and of the maintenance of quality through a sort of pyramidal set of hierarchies extending nationwide to communities and physicians' offices, with apices in the relevant sections of academic medical centers. The research imperative, however, also bears responsibility for many of the system's problems for it is motivated by the question: "What can be done?" That something has not been previously discovered, developed, or perfected is sufficient reason for pursuing an investigation, possibly even in the face of serious doubts about the likelihood of socially useful or moral outcomes. The extension of the research imperative to clinical medicine seems often to have substituted prolongation and saving of life for relief

99

of suffering as the primary ethical medical responsibility. The relentless technological extension of life of doomed patients of all ages is not only of little permanent value, but such prolongation of pain and suffering is a dramatically critical factor in the dangerous escalation of medical costs.

The research imperative asks, "What *can* be done?" The ethicist or moral philosopher asks, "What, all things considered, *ought* to be done?"[44] The answering of this question is the task of the institutional committee considering the social and moral suitability of a grant application for a university. It is also the task of the hospital ethics committee as it attempts to deal with ethical dilmemmas occurring in the medical care of seriously ill patients.

With the advent of "big science," such as the space telescope and the huge new linear accelerator, there may well have been too little consideration of the effect of such hugely expensive enterprises on the funding of individual basic research, and on their impact on creative scientific thought in general. Technology and knowledge exist for their development—therefore proceed! The same "Can it be done?" question appears to have been answered affirmatively for the Human Genome project.[45] It is under way, with funding apparently guaranteed from both NIH and the Department of Energy (DOE), in spite of the opposition of many medical scientists who are not only skeptical of the ultimate value that might accrue from the project, but who are also deeply concerned about its impact on individual investigators who have been the core of our scientific advances. It is true that medical ethics is represented on the planning group for the Human Genome project, and that some attention will be given not only to the ethical validity of the project itself, but also to some of the powerful implications of its results vis-à-vis human manipulation and some of the very basic issues implied in its subject matter for human dignity and freedom.

NOTES

1. Thomas N. Bonner, *American Doctors and German Universities: A Chapter in Internatational Intellectual Relations 1870–1914* (Lincoln: University of Nebraska Press, 1963).
2. Two of the main investigators of the period in Germany were Richard Koch and Robert Virchow. Koch (1843–1910), a founder of bacteriology, invented solid culture plates and specific stains, discovered the tubercle bacillus, and won the Nobel Prize in 1905. Virchow (1821–1902), was professor of Anatomy at Wurzburg in 1846. He worked with tumors, concentrated on cell pathology, and wrote "Pathology of Tumors" in 1862.
3. See, for example, the following *JAMA* issues, which carry extensive minutes of meetings of the Council on Medical Education chaired by Dr. Arthur D. Bevan. Both issues discuss the advisability of higher standards of admission, more language requirements, and the importance of stiffer licensing laws because the number of medical schools was clearly too large, etc.: *JAMA* 44, no. 18 (1905): 1470–75; and *JAMA* 48, no. 20 (1907): 1701–7.
4. Kenneth M. Ludmerer, *Learning to Heal: The Development of American Medical Education* (New York: Basic Books, Inc., 1985), 47–71.
5. Donald Fleming, *William H. Welch and the Rise of Modern Medicine* (Baltimore: The Johns Hopkins University Press, 1987).
6. A. M. Chesney, *The Johns Hopkins Hospital and The Johns Hopkins School of Medicine: A Chronicle*, vol. 1 (Baltimore: The Johns Hopkins University Press, 1943).
7. Richard H. Shyrock, *American Medical Research* (New York: The Commonwealth Fund, 1947). Much of this section on research during the early period of American medical education is taken from this work.
8. Thomas Parran, *The Aims of the Public Health Service,* Smithsonian Institution Annual Report, 1937 (Washington, D.C.: Government Printing Office, 1938), 463 ff., 464.
9. P.L. 75–244.
10. United States Senate, Committee on Military Affairs, *Report from the Subcommittee on War Mobilization on Wartime Research and Development,* 1940–44, pt. 1: vii.
11. F. D. Roosevelt, "Letter on the Office of Scientific Research and Development," *Science* 100 (1944): 542.
12. Vannevar Bush, *Science, the Endless Frontier: A Report to the President on a Program for Postwar Scientific Research,* July, 1945. (Reprinted, Washington, D.C.: National Science Foundation, 1960).
13. Ibid., 15.
14. Ibid.
15. Stephen P. Strickland, *Politics, Science, and Dread Disease: A Short History of United States Medical Research Policy* (Cambridge: Harvard University Press, 1972), 29.
16. Ibid., 29–30.
17. Ibid., 32.
18. Ibid., 35.
19. Ibid., 37.
20. The following are examples of citations about Great Society Programs: R. Q. Marston, et al., "Regional Medical Programs: A Progress Report," *American Journal of Public Health* 58 (1968): 726–30; M. E. Odoroff,

"Measuring Progress of Regional Medical Programs," *American Journal of Public Health* 58 (1968): 726–30; and D. C. Schnauss, "Comprehensive Health Planning: A Boon or a Bane?" *Hospital Programs* (48 (1967): 63–67.

21. At the time of Shannon's appointment, the NIH consisted of the National Cancer Institute, the National Heart Institute, the National Institute of Dental Research, the National Institute of Neurological Diseases and Blindness, the National Institute of Arthritis and Metabolic Diseases, and the National Institute of Allergy and Infectious Diseases. Later were formed the National Institute of General Medical Sciences (1963); the National Institute for Child Health and Human Development (1963); the National Eye Institute, with NINDB renamed the National Institute of Neurological Diseases and Stroke (1968). In 1969 the NHI was renamed the National Heart and Lung Institute, and the National Institute for Environmental Health Sciences was established within Research Triangle Park, N.C. in 1972. Blood was added to the name of the National Heart and Lung Institute, resulting in the new name, National Heart, Lung, and Blood Institute. The National Institute on Aging was founded in 1974; in 1980 the name of the NIAMD was changed to the National Institute of Arthritis, Diabetes, and Digestive and Kidney Diseases. In 1985, the National Institute of Arthritis and Musculoskeletal and Skin Diseases was founded.

22. U.S. Deptartment of Health and Human Services, *1987 NIH Almanac*, NIH Publication no. 87–5, September 1987.

23. J. R. Schofield, *New and Expanded Medical Schools, Mid-Century to the 1980s* (San Francisco: Jossey-Bass Publishers, 1984), 21.

24. Ibid., 19–28, for more discussion of these legislative actions. Also see the table on pp. 24–25 summarizing the events of this period.

25. Vernon W. Lippard, *A Half Century of American Medical Education, 1920–1970* (New York: Macy Foundation, 1974).

26. George E. Miller, et al., *Teaching and Learning in Medical School* (Cambridge: Harvard University Press, The Commonwealth Fund, 1961).

27. Edward Shorter, *The Health Century* (New York: Doubleday, 1987), 93.

28. James B. Wyngaarden, "A Century of Science for Health." *Clinical Research* 1988; January, 36(1):3–4.

29. Ludmerer, 264.

30. William G. Rothstein, *American Medical Schools and the Practice of Medicine, a History* (New York: Oxford University Press, 1987), 257.

31. AAMC Institutional Profile System Ranking Report. Run on 11/06/87. Request 2015: Research Expenditures.

32. *Research Activity of Full-Time Faculty in Departments of Medicine* (Washington, D.C.: APM and AAMC, 1987).

33. Ibid., 38.

34. Ibid., 46.

35. *Higher Education and the Nation's Health. Policies for Medical and Dental Education,* a special report and recommendations by the Carnegie Commission on Higher Education (New York: McGraw-Hill Book Company, 1970).

36. Ibid,. 73.

37. Ibid., 70–71.

38. *Progress and Problems in Medical and Dental Education: Federal Support Versus Federal Control*, a report of the Carnegie Council on Policy Studies in Higher Education (San Francisco: Jossey-Bass, 1976).

39. John A. D. Cooper, "The Association of American Medical Colleges: Looking Ahead from the First Hundred Years," *Journal of Medical Education* 52 (1977): 11–19.

40. H. S. Barrows, "The Tutorial Process," *Southern Illinois University School of Medicine* (1989), 43.

41. *The New York Times*, February 28, 1988, E-5.

42. *Florida Times-Union* (Jacksonville), December 14, 1989.

43. AAMC, *Washington D.C. Weekly Report* 3, no. 42, (1989).

44. This is covered in most books on ethics. For me a useful and clear explication of this position, see Martin Benjamin and Joy Curtis, *Ethics in Nursing* (London: Oxford University Press, 1981), 10.

45. J. D. Watson, "The Human Genome Project: Past, Present, and Future," *Science* 248 (1990): 44–49.

5
Accreditation of Medical Schools

THE NATURE OF ACCREDITATION

Accreditation of educational institutions is a process which generally has been delegated by the public to the relevant professional establishment. While state and federal governments are interested observers in the accreditation process, their involvement is usually minimal except in the matter of ascertaining the existence of acceptable institutional standards for the receipt of federal research funds. We have seen how the great revolution in medical education in the early 1900s included Flexner's powerful recommendations for the inclusion of medical education within the structure of universities, with issues such as curriculum development, academic structure, and faculty salaries governed by the greater university. We have also noted the critical roles of such universities as Harvard, Pennsylvania, Michigan, and Johns Hopkins in this process. We have described the original Coggeshall recommendations and their plea for the AAMC to reorganize itself so as to recognize the subordinate role of the medical school within the domain of higher education. The rejection of some of these recommendations appears to have aided the growth of the AAMC as an organization that tends to operate independently of parent universities. Accreditation is the predominant tool by which the AAMC and AMA influence and control medical school educational and organizational policy. This partnership, in the context of the Liaison Committee on Medical Education, further appears to accentuate the separation of medical education from its often stated closeness with higher education in general. The following will investigate the nature of the relationship between accreditation of medical schools and the process by which similar certification is bestowed on the universities themselves.

GENERAL UNIVERSITY ACCREDITATION

In their accreditation process, universities are generally surveyed by regional organizations such as the North Central

Association of Colleges and Schools or the Committee on Institutional Cooperation (CIC), a consortium of the Big Ten Universities plus the University of Chicago. The CIC Statement of Principles of Accreditation is a carefully worded document that considers the constraints, limitations, and mutual advantages of the accrediting process that these universities find relevant to themselves, and is probably representative of the attitudes of universities in general. I have selected sections from this statement of principles that seem to stand in contrast to similar guidelines which form the basis for medical school accreditation. The pertinence of this document to our discussion would seem clear, since several CIC universities have medical schools accredited by the LCME.[1] In all probability, they reflect the general attitude of institutions of higher education on this subject. The following selections from this document seem to me to be relevant to the issue of medical school accreditation; my comments are appended.

1. Evaluation must place its emphasis on the outcome of the educational process. "Criticisms by accrediting teams directed at procedural or organizational details must be based on reasonable evidence that those details affect the performance of graduates or the quality of education provided to them."

This principle seems at odds with the experience of some medical schools who feel they have been pressured by their accreditation agency into modifying projected administrative innovations or curricular departures from the norm, or including such extramural examinations as the National Boards as measures of curricular validity.

2. The standards applied in the accreditation process must not discourage experimentation, innovation or modernization, either in teaching methods or in the curriculum itself. What an accrediting body "must not do is impose standards that place obstacles in the way of originality, creativity, or innovation on the part of the faculty or the institution."

The university, then, should seek appropriate creative and innovative ways to go about the management and modification of educational processes as relevant to achieving institutional goals and objectives. The mandate to accrediting bodies does not include forcing the elimination of such efforts, even in the face of uncertainty about ultimate success of the innovation.

4. The accreditation report must explicitly recognize institutional diversity. "Every university has its own unique resources, methodologies, special mission, and educational philosophy.... Each university can expect that accrediting teams

will familiarize themselves with its special circumstances and resources and will take them into account in relation to the programs being reviewed."

The idea, then, that each medical school must be structured as a semiautonomous institute, with structure and function conforming to extramurally and professionally mandated standards, is questionable if medical education is to be considered an integral part of higher education.

5. Accreditation should not encourage the isolation or self-containment of an Academic Program. "A university can expect an accrediting team to file a report that shows awareness of these supporting resources and actively encourages their shared use."

The tendency has existed for the LCME to ignore such situations and to press for duplication within the medical school setting.

8. In the case of professional schools, although there must be significant input from the profession itself, the ultimate authority over educational policies must remain firmly in the hands of the academic community.

This principle recognizes the responsibility resting with the profession to have appropriate input to the program, but insists that the ultimate responsibility must reside with the university. Once again, the institution is ultimately responsible for the quality of the program.

Thus, the CIC's set of principles concerning accreditation specifically asserts the primacy of the university for all its educational programs. It emphasizes the need for universities to cooperate with professional accreditation bodies, and the need to recognize the significant contributions of the professions in assuring that student learning is compatible with professional standards. The basic concerns of professional accreditors should be educational outcomes rather than instructional or organizational details. The accrediting body should not intrude itself into valid educational innovations, the operation of which is part and parcel of the university's obligation to society.

THE LCME AND MEDICAL SCHOOL ACCREDITATION

It should be remembered that from the beginnings of the medical educational revolution in the early 1900s, the pleas of Flexner and other educators notwithstanding, the burden of establishing the standards of medical education was assumed by the medical profession as its own particular area of responsibility. I was recently accorded the courtesy of a meeting with the AMA's accreditation staff in the organization's headquarters, and permitted to tape the proceedings.[2] This group was well informed on the history of medical school accreditation, and was most generous with both their time and the degree to which they openly discussed important issues. The following is a summary of that meeting.

The role of the AMA's Council on Medical Education in the early twentieth century and its emphasis on curriculum details was emphasized, even to the point of specifying the required teaching hours for the basic and clinical sciences. Figured into their deliberations were the pass-fail rates of graduates on state board examinations. The Council on Medical Education published its first list of approved schools in 1907 and continued periodically thereafter to survey medical schools. An "A-B-C" classification of medical schools was developed with "A" being satisfactory, "B" unsatisfactory but with potential for improvement, and "C" incurable or hopeless. The AAMC had been visiting medical schools even before the AMA had begun this process, resulting in a period during which schools were surveyed by both organizations. Their 1942 convergence under the LCME umbrella initiated joint surveys, with both the AAMC and AMA reserving to themselves the responsibility for making independent evaluations and recommendations. It was not until the early 1970s that both parties agreed that such matters as putting schools on probation, removing probationary status, or withdrawing accreditation should be delegated to the LCME whose decisions were to be absolutely final and independent of review. There have been disagreements with the organization of university presidents who were supporting regional versus professional accrediting bodies. Such strife at one time had been particularly acute in New York State, which had established its own regional accrediting body, raising some question about the validity there of the professional accrediting processes. The tension between professional, governmental, and general university prerogatives vis-à-vis accreditation, while still present, seems for now to have been at least temporarily resolved. The feeling was that serious differences had been worked out between most specialized programs and the various regional accrediting agencies. In connection with the discussion of relationships between the LCME and the regional accrediting bodies, the point was made in this meeting that the LCME accredits only programs within institutions that lead to the MD degree—not total institutions. An effort is currently being made to coordinate LCME visits with those of regional agencies; one such coordinated institutional visit was currently being planned.

The group seemed ambivalent about the true status of accreditation of medical schools by the LCME. While the process was stated to be a voluntary one, nonetheless the power of the LCME to pass final judgment on the very existence of medical schools was also clearly stated. Professional control of the accreditation process seemed to achieve legal status at the state level early in this century with the recognition by state licensing boards of schools approved either by the AAMC, or more commonly by the AMA Council on Medical Education and Hospitals.

Federal interest in medical school accreditation developed from the problems engendered by returning World War II veterans who were seeking governmental tuition benefits under the GI Bill. To the government there seemed to be little difference between occupational training programs and professional education programs. The multitude of these programs increased the bureaucratic power of the United States Office of Education, which developed rigid criteria for recognizing an accrediting body. The resultant need for periodic petitions by the LCME for renewal of recognition became a cumbersome and expensive activity which continues to this time, although its adversarial nature has been somewhat modified.

The controlling membership on the LCME is held by the AAMC and the AMA, each of whom selects six members. The AAMC members are selected by the Executive Council. The AMA process is centralized in its Board of Trustees, which appoints members upon recommendation by the Council on Medical Education and Hospitals. The LCME itself selects two public members, two student members who are elected by the respective student groups, and a Canadian member representing that country's medical school accrediting body, the CACMS. A representative from the federal Office of Education is usually present at meetings. It was emphasized to me that the public members, not being expert in the field of medical education, are in a position to temper the twelve professional members, who may express strong feelings about liberal or conservative sides of given issues.

The recommendations for public representation originated with the Office of Education because representatives of consumer groups at one or two hearings had expressed the opinion that accreditation should be a public responsibility. (They likened a profession-dominated process to a "fox guarding a henhouse.") The addition of public members seemed a good compromise between the apparent absurdity of a totally public-dominated process and one which, while having clear public implications, requires leadership from those with intensive professional and academic expertise. The group was unanimous in feeling that the public members had brought a new perspective to the LCME.

During the 1960s, after the AAMC's move to Washington D.C. and coincidentally with its appointment of a new LCME staff director, the accreditation process seemed to take on new vigor. This was also the beginning of the period in which several new medical schools were in early stages of planning or development. Encouraged by favorable federal legislation and by such sources as the Kellogg Foundation with its program of funding two-year medical schools, several universities contemplated expansion into medical education. Some of these institutions—especially those located on Caribbean islands—had questionable resources and comprehension of the ultimate costs or complexities of such education. Hence, appropriately, the LCME appeared to be surveying these new schools with a fervor not customarily applied to established institutions. My meeting in the AMA offices revealed some of the dilemmas faced by the LCME during this period. This plethora of potential new schools put an almost unmanageable burden on both staff and LCME members. It also seemed apparent that some of the proposed new schools were neither well conceived nor endowed with knowledgeable leadership. As requests came to the LCME to enter the accreditation cycle, some proposals, classified as "exciting experiments in medical education," appeared to LCME members to lack precise protocol and to be devoid of plans or criteria for measuring results.

While the story of the diffusion of new educational research findings into new programs and fledgling medical schools has been told in chapter 3, a short recapitulation here has relevance to the issues these changes posed for the LCME during the 1960s and 1970s. It will be recalled that the first major effort to alter the medical curriculum had occurred at Western Reserve University during the 1950s. Its features included early clinical experiences, group learning of the basic sciences, emphasis on interdepartmental collaboration, and clinical relevance of the sciences. Assisted in this effort by the Commonwealth Fund, it was the subject of a number of publications.[3] The 1960s and 1970s, with strong AAMC support, saw the flourishing of research in medical education. With George Miller one of its leaders, great emphasis was placed on the introduction of general educational principles and methods into teaching and learning in the basic and clinical sciences of medicine.[4] Federal money became available to help with these projects. Some basic work was sponsored by the AAMC, and its annual meeting began to feature a section on Research in Medical Education (RIME). The upshot of all of this was the recognition of basic flaws in traditional teaching techniques such as reliance on lectures, rote learning, and "cookbook" laboratory exercises. Demonstration programs, often developed by faculty heavily involved in medical education research, were beginning to suggest alternative teaching methods characterized by such features as an emphasis on clinical relevance, student self-learning, and faculty-led group process as basic principles of physician education. Faculty members, attracted to this new wave of academic endeavor, looked to some of the new schools as promising sites for the introduction of these new techniques. The new curricula developed in such situations sometimes required administrative innovation. Thus, standards for appointment and promotion were modified, as were the responsibilities of department chairpersons; departments (or other administrative units) of medical education appeared; and allocation of considerable money for implementation of the interdisciplinary parts of the programs became necessary. Inevitably, some of these methods were controversial with both the conservative members of the faculties of the innovative schools and many LCME members, who tended to be drawn from research-rich traditional institutions.

A further problem for the LCME was that the federal government needed a "Letter of Reasonable Assurance" that the new school had a reasonable chance of succeeding, in order for it to qualify for government funds for construction, program, or research grants. A new institution, therefore, whose plans were devoid of risk—and generally hewed the traditional educational mode—had less difficulty receiving such a go-ahead than did one with innovative and possibly untried administrative and curricular arrangements.

In this connection it was not uncommon for difficulty to develop within the accrediting process itself. During the four days of extensive discussion normally spent with faculty, administrators, and students of the school being investigated, the visiting team could sometimes be convinced of the validity of an innovative program and become enthusiastic and optimistic as to subsequent LCME action. A month or two later, the school might be acutely disappointed by a major reversal of the team's report after consideration by the LCME in its official meeting. Such unexpected outcomes then lead to burdensome appeals by the deans which could culminate in special appearances before the LCME. Reversals of unfavorable accreditation decisions sometimes result.

In chapter 2 we discussed the issue of National Board examinations, particularly Part I, as a disturbing factor in the new medical school-LCME relationship. The official position of the LCME is that it has never had a stipulation that National Boards be required as evaluation instruments in all medical schools. With many new schools, however, especially those with apparently untried educational or administrative programs, the LCME feels that an external evaluation of the learning effectiveness of such programs would prove or disprove their efficacy. With the absence of any acceptable alternative external examination, some schools were, in effect, forced to adopt a policy requiring students to take National Board, Part I examinations before proceeding to the clinical years. Failure to comply would have had serious accreditational consequences. The position of the LCME has been that its primary purpose is to protect the public from inadequately prepared physicians; National Boards seem the best available guideline for relevant educational success. Stimulating innovation in the interest of improved medical educational outcomes was considered, at best, a secondary objective.

In the past, the LCME has had a sort of grading system for institutional accreditation, with length of term of accreditation being the relevant variable. Thus, accreditation would be awarded for 1, 3, or 10 years, with the length of the award considered a measure of degree of approval. This procedure often resulted in dissatisfaction on the part of the schools, based on invidious comparisons, jealousies, and antagonisms between the schools themselves and increased tension with the LCME. Recently, the variable level of approval has been replaced by a standard seven-year period of accreditation. This, however, does not free a questionable school from interim visits or requirements for periodic progress reports. During the seventh year of accreditation and before the official visit, the schools themselves carry out an intense self-study according to guidelines provided by the LCME.

Current procedure also includes a review of the survey teams' reports by about sixty outside reviewers who are polled prior to review by the LCME. These reviewers are culled from a population of deans, associate deans, and others familiar with medical education who are asked to comment on the appropriateness and fairness of survey teams' recommendations.

Thus, the LCME itself, with assistance from its AAMC and AMA staffs, feels that it has developed a fair and effective method for the implementation of its mission to guarantee institutional maintenance of high standards of teaching and scholarly productivity, and for assuring the public that graduates of American medical schools are of high quality. The focus of LCME accreditation activity has become a document specifying approved standards for medical school structure and function.

FUNCTIONS AND STRUCTURE OF A MEDICAL SCHOOL STANDARDS FOR ACCREDITATION OF MEDICAL EDUCATION PROGRAMS LEADING TO THE M.D. DEGREE[5]

This document, periodically revised by the AMA and the AAMC governing bodies, is the "bible" of the accreditation process. It provides guidelines designed to assure uniform applicability and due process for the accreditation of all medical schools. It is read by team members, and by administrators and key faculty of the schools being visited. The document, while essentially objective and declarative of support for such values as the instillation of "lifelong habits of learning, dedication to service, and the values and attitudes consistent with a compassionate profession,"[6] seems to be based on criteria most comfortably applicable to the complete modern academic medical center with a full panoply of departments and residency-training programs. For example, we find in the introduction that

> ... the LCME considers it vital for the education of medical students that each school provide, or be affiliated with institutions that provide programs in graduate medical education (residencies) and that

112

the faculty of each school actively contributes to the development and transmission of new knowledge.

In response to current expansion of the definition of scholarly activity it does, however, state,

In addition to biologically oriented studies, research investigations may include, among others, the cultural and behavioral aspects of medicine, methods for provision of medical care, and the process of medical education.

On page 6, the introduction states:

The accreditation status of programs leading to the M.D. degree is determined solely by the Liaison Committee on Medical Education. To be accredited, programs must meet the national standards set forth in this document as judged by the LCME. These standards are sometimes stated in a fashion that is not susceptible to quantification or to precise definition because the nature of the evaluation is qualitative in character and can be accomplished only by the exercise of professional judgment by qualified persons.

The introduction goes on to elucidate the document's use of the words "must" and "should."

Use of the word "must" indicates that the LCME considers meeting the standard to be absolutely necessary if the program is to be accredited. Use of the word "should" indicates that the LCME considers an attribute to be highly desirable and makes a judgment as to whether or not its absence may compromise substantial compliance with all of the requirements for accreditation.

It is further stated that the standards for accreditation are developed through a process of study and debate, including public hearings. A standing committee of the LCME is charged with the ongoing evaluation of standards, changes in which must be approved by the AAMC's Executive Council and the AMA's Council on Medical Education, and by appropriate Canadian counterparts. The various levels of accreditation are described: provisional accreditation for new schools and full accreditation for established schools or those with earlier provisional accreditation; or, full or provisional accreditation may be denied, a school may be put on probation, or accreditation may be withdrawn.

It is difficult to take exception to the statements in the section entitled "Educational Program," most of which verge on the obvious for a field as well defined as the basic structure of medical education. One can, however, become interested in the "must-should" dichotomy. For example, we find that the program of education *must* include at least 130 weeks of instruction. The program *must* "be designed to provide a general professional education, recognizing that, this alone, is insufficient to prepare a graduate for independent, unsupervised practice." While the faculty is responsible for the design, implementation, and evaluation of the curriculum (presumably a "must"), a committee of this faculty *should* do this work with support of the chief executive officer and staff. An entire paragraph on the committee responsible for curriculum is couched in "shoulds," including giving "careful attention to the impact on students of the amount of work required." It should "monitor the content provided in each discipline in order that objectives for education of a physician are achieved without attempting to present the complete, detailed, systematic body of knowledge in that discipline. The objectives, content, and methods of pedagogy utilized for each segment of the curriculum, as well as for the entire curriculum, likewise, should be subjected to periodic evaluation."

Ambiguities are apparent for both the personnel of the school seeking accreditation and education-oriented LCME members. Does not, for example, the provision of a "general professional education" (as opposed to "training") include protection against deleterious overwork on the part of students? Does it not protect the student against an overzealous faculty member who might push students to master all the anatomy of the human body? Does it not assume as a "must" the periodic evaluation of curricular objectives? Indeed, a pedagogically-oriented faculty believing in the value of process over content might well establish these "shoulds" as "musts," allowing detailed content to emerge as an almost secondary value.

Similar possibilities for confusion are apparent in the section on "Content." There seems little ambiguity in the statement of faculty responsibility for devising

> ... a curriculum that permits the student to learn the fundamental principles of medicine, to acquire skills of critical judgment based on evidence and experience, and to develop an ability to use principles and skills wisely in solving problems of health and disease.

This is couched in terms suggesting "must," and would seem to be adequate as a general set of guidelines. In the next sentence, however, we find that

> ... the curriculum must be designed so that students acquire an understanding of the scientific concepts underlying medicine. In designing the curriculum, the faculty must introduce current advances in the basic and clinical sciences, including therapy and technology, changes in the understanding of disease, and the effect of social needs and demands on medical care.

While it cannot be all-encompassing, the curriculum "must include the sciences basic to medicine, a variety of clinical disciplines, and ethical, behavioral, and socioeconomic subjects pertinent to medicine. There should be presentation of material on medical ethics and human values." Medical ethics, therefore, is both "must" and "should." In view of the ambivalence with which this subject is regarded by many physicians and educators, this may be appropriate.

It is my feeling that the *should-must* verbiage of these paragraphs might well be modified so as to eliminate confusion and ambivalence. Were many of the *shoulds* to be recognized as essential to quality, student-oriented learning, this section could be converted into one recognizing the validity of both "traditional" and "progressive" educational features.

By and large, though, the document is a clear statement of standards by which medical schools may be judged. However, this document does not always seem to be the main standard for medical school accreditation. Particularly liable to criticism and negative LCME action have been programs in new schools which, for example, put a high value on community settings as learning sites, particularly during the preclinical years. Nowhere in the document can be found a reference to the necessity for external examinations to measure student progress or to evaluate the efficacy of the educational program. Yet accreditation of some schools has been held hostage to the requirement of National Board examinations for students. Furthermore, even in some new schools in which the National Board requirement has been adopted, accreditation has been withheld pending achievement of some sort of national test score standard.

The guidelines suggest that curriculum and its evaluation are the areas about which most controversy currently rages. One factor in this seemingly interminable debate is the perceived threat to basic science departments contained within modern self-learning educational theories and programs. Since an apparent downgrading of the volume of content in these subjects tends to be part of such educational programs, understandable fear of loss of funds and status motivates the academic resistance to curricula based on these educational concepts. Therefore, when such alterations in the traditional staffing pattern for medical student education are contemplated, part of the management role is to negotiate with the departments in a way that clarifies departmental goals and objectives vis-à-vis those of the institution. Thus, a department of anatomy that trains graduate students and does productive research might not necessarily need to accept smaller budgets if institutional goals include Ph.D training and research productivity. Furthermore, teaching in the context of small group self-learning, although perhaps requiring less of the faculty member's specific knowledge, is equally valuable to the M.D. educational program. It has been my experience, both at Michigan State and now at Mercer, that prominent basic science investigators, once they have experienced participation in problem-based learning, often become converts and enthusiastic supporters.

LEGAL ASPECTS OF MEDICAL SCHOOL ACCREDITATION

The LCME guidelines specify the close link between medical education and the nature of private medical practice. The dominant stated purpose of medical education and residency training is to prepare the student ultimately for "independent, unsupervised practice." This emphasis on independence and lack of supervision is in accord with the profession's notion of the ideal status of the physician in society—namely, to be one's own boss in one's own setting, encumbered by a minimum of outside influence on the quality, style, or cost of what one does. Under antitrust law, such a practice-cum-small-business must compete, rather than cooperate, with other medical practitioners in the same community. This may well have come as a surprise to those who have faced federal prosecution for having tried to work with colleagues in efforts to develop such presumably socially beneficent goals as communitywide fees for given services. It is not surprising that the profession-managed accrediting process for this system might be vulnerable to similar federal attention.

The legal implications of the accreditation process have been described by a number of authors, particularly Havighurst, who deals expressly with the antitrust perspective of such private and voluntary accreditation.[7] The basic position of his analysis is that voluntary accreditation of private programs should in no way inhibit the normal competitiveness of such systems. In general, the articles emphasize what we already know: that the medical profession is monolithic in its behavior and that the credentialing systems, whether dealing with the basic education of physicians in medical schools or certification of specialists, serves to reenforce this state of affairs.

According to the provisions of the Sherman Antitrust Act, the Federal Trade Commission, which monitors the field of private competitive businesses, should be the agency that interprets medical school accrediting activity. However, the author states that

> So far, the FTC has taken few actions with respect to credentialing and accrediting in the health care field. In 1977, the FTC staff opposed, with limited success, the U.S.Commissioner of Education and the LCME as accreditor of medical schools; the issue raised was the AMA's heavy involvement in the LCME and the possibility that this involvement enabled the medical profession to exercise undue influence over the number of physicians being trained.[8]

At that time it was possible that a complaint might be brought against the American Board of Plastic Surgery, because board-

116

certified otolaryngologists were as well qualified as plastic surgeons to perform certain facial plastic surgery. This was not pursued because of the notion that differences of opinion concerning certification's value should be resolved in the marketplace, rather than in an antitrust court or regulatory tribunal.

Throughout Part II, the authors belabor the essentially monopolistic nature of American medicine. For example,

> Unfortunately, competition in health services has not focused enough on values, preferences, costs, or alternative ideas about how health needs should be met. Instead, because of the dominance of a single-profession-sponsored-ideology, health care competition has concentrated primarily on the amenities surrounding the provision of an essentially uniform product. Although the American health care system is certainly the most pluralistic in the world, it still reflects the strong preference of organized professional groups for centralizing decision making on important issues in professional hands. (265)

In other words, they see the continuation of the AMA's nineteenth-century policy of medical practice as private enterprise as a serious complication vis-à-vis medical education within the setting of the university.

Among the most cherished notions of the medical profession is the recurrent declaration of the patient's "free choice of physician"—in itself a lullaby justifying the present system.

> The most intricate and complete mechanism for standardizing system inputs is that governing the training and labeling of personnel produced for service in the system. . . . Although it can be argued that unlimited proliferation of health care options would endanger ignorant consumers and raise the cost of searching the market, there is good reason to believe that standardization has prevented desirable competition. Many options potentially attractive to rational health care consumers have been effectively foreclosed by professional bodies exercising formal and informal powers over educational and other institutions and over individual providers. Although consumers can choose among a large number of competing practitioners, the medical profession has sought to confine consumers, as much as possible, to choose among things which in the most crucial respects do not significantly differ. Thus, the consumer's "free choice of physician," so jealously guarded by professional interests through the years, has implied very limited freedom to choose anything but a physician. Moreover, aside from osteopaths and a few foreign medical graduates who have leaded [sic] into the system, the options available to consumers exercising free choice of physician have included only the relatively homogeneous products of a controlled education process. (267–68)

The gist of these articles, then, is that the systems of accreditation of the medical schools and of the certification of individuals as specialists have become one of the effective means for control over who becomes a physician, and who becomes a specialist. Furthermore, the system of accrediting hospitals, by the Joint Commission on the Accreditation of Hospitals (JCAH), composed as it is of members of the specialties of medicine—to wit the AMA, the American Hospital Association, the American College of Physicians, and the American College of Surgeons—seems to be composed of people of identical philosophical stripe. That these branches of the health professions frequently disagree on policies relating to hospital accreditation is predictable.

> Although intraprofessional debates occur over standards, the four sponsors have agreed among themselves not to express their separate views for the benefit of consumers and instead to arrive at and abide by a common position expressed through the JCAH. A joint venture eliminating competition among the four dominant firms in any industry is normally subject to the closest antitrust scrutiny, and probably not even compelling proof of scale economies could overcome the presumption against such collaborations. There is no apparent reason why this principle should not apply to a joint venture to accredit hospitals. (323–24)

In summary, then, legal analysis suggests that the accreditation mechanisms for most of the health professions appear to have been influential in inhibiting competition between individuals, hospitals, and other health care arrangements. With medical care generally having assumed the mode of private practice, and with a Supreme Court declaration that medicine was subject to the Sherman Act, it has found itself to be increasingly under the same legal constraints as business. With the AMA sharing equally the organizational responsibility for staffing and operating the LCME, the validity of American medicine's educational accreditation process remains legally ambiguous.

Presumably this problem will ultimately be resolved. Relevant information is not readily available, and predictions of outcome are certainly inappropriate. One could speculate, however, that the existence and utilization of a common standard such as the "Functions and Structure of a Medical School" for accreditation purposes seriously limits competition between medical schools, and inhibits their participation in experimental curricular or patient care initiatives. While promoting sound and modern medical care, a dependence on research developments as the foundation of medical knowledge can automatically militate against teaching competing theories of etiology and treatment which, at times, may be relevant when working with populations of ethnic minorities. The inevitable relationship between research findings and high technology, furthermore, tends to place a higher value on greater specialized medicine than on the less technologically sophisticated activities of primary care and family practice.

ACCREDITATION AND THE NEW MEDICAL SCHOOLS

The procedure employed by a university actively seeking to expand into the field of medical education is to request an informal survey by the LCME. Presumably, by then, the institution has established the general fashion in which the new school will be funded. In the case of a state university, it probably has some sort of go-ahead from the legislature, and plans for recruiting faculty and for the acquisition of space for both preclinical teaching and clinical work. A preliminary visit by AMA or AAMC staff members has generally been helpful in estimating probabilities of success, and understanding the subsequent procedures in the accreditation process. These include a request that the LCME write a "Letter of Reasonable Assurance" to the federal government before the first class is admitted in order to qualify the school to apply for any sort of federal aid. The next step is provisional accreditation. On page 6, the "Functions and Structure of a Medical School" states: "For a program to be considered for evaluation for initial provisional accreditation, the school must submit documentation that its proposed program can be expected to meet the standards for accreditation by the time that the projected number of first-year students is admitted." After review and acceptance of the documents, the LCME makes a determination of the readiness for the scheduling of a survey team visit. Based on the completed presurvey data base questionnaire, the report of the survey team, and the comments of a panel appointed to review the report, the LCME determines whether or not to award provisional accreditation. "Once provisionally accredited, a school is reevaluated annually for continued provisional accreditation in similar fashion until the year of graduation of the charter class." Prior to this, the school completes an institutional self-study in addition to developing an extensive data base, the materials and forms for which are provided by the LCME. "Based on consideration of the data base, self-study, and findings of the survey, the LCME decides whether or not to award initial full accreditation."

Periodic LCME revisits are then scheduled according to previously determined schedules. Formerly, full accreditation was awarded for varying periods of time according the LCME estimates of the degree to which the new school had succeeded. Now, however, there is but one standard seven-year term of accreditation. This may well be adequate at a time when few, if any, new schools are being developed. Some of us who led new schools during the 1960s and 1970s, however, look back with mixed feelings about the accreditation process for developing schools. While the experience was uniformly interesting and informative, with team members generally being distinguished academicians and often good friends, the intensity of the effort required to prepare for visits seemed distracting and inordinately demanding of valuable faculty and administrative time. The anxiety generated by these visits, especially if stressful criticism or even denigration of the validity of some program feature emerged, could seriously dampen faculty and student morale. Even in cases when the visiting team was favorably impressed and encouraging during its final report to the dean and the university president, a reversal of the tentative positive report by the LCME at its next meeting was entirely possible. The following are summaries of accreditation experiences of two medical schools which originated during the past twenty-five years, and with which I have been closely associated: Michigan State University College of Human Medicine and Mercer University School of Medicine.

MICHIGAN STATE UNIVERSITY

Our initial experience at Michigan State with accreditation was essentially the same as at other contemporary new schools, namely, that the early phases of the process were helpful. Staff members were generally fair and encouraging, yet appropriately skeptical about contemplated innovations. For example, my July 1964 appointment as dean was interpreted by the university president as a mandate to admit the first class in the fall of 1965. This schedule was clearly impossible. The problem was resolved only after a one-year postponement was demanded by the LCME. Early LCME visits provided the opportunity to explain the proposed administrative innovations by which all-university basic science departments, already shared by Veterinary Medicine and other colleges, would be shared by Human Medicine as well. Also described, but only weakly supported, was the notion that our involvement within a huge state university commanding magnificent resources would permit close relationships with behavioral science and humanities departments, and with the College of Education. The partnership with Veterinary Medicine, furthermore, might emerge as a potent stimulus for comparative biological and behavioral research.

In addition to the recurrent incredulity by site visitors about the feasibility of deanly "control" over shared science departments, the problems that developed included our notion of a central interdisciplinary "core" of human biology to be run concurrently with more traditional departmental offerings; the later development of the "focal problem" approach to student learning; the utilization of community hospitals for the required clinical learning experiences; the Upper Peninsula Program; and, finally, our resistance to pressure to require National Board, Part I examinations as a nationally valid measure of student progress and of curricular adequacy.

Shared Departments

With departments of anatomy, biochemistry, microbiology, pathology, pharmacology, and physiology already well developed and productive in research, the university's central administration saw little logic in duplicating administrative units for Human Medicine. Rather, as with Agriculture, Natural Science, and Veterinary Medicine, these units would simply be shared by the new medical college. Needed incremental funding for relevant faculty positions would be incorporated in the new college's annual budget requests. In practice, the LCME's concern about inadequate control by the medical dean did not turn out to be a significant problem; negotiations with the other relevant deans were usually amicable. Indeed, the size of some of these departments insured a considerably larger research base than would otherwise have been possible. Some resistance developed, however, in enlisting cooperation for staffing of our various interdisciplinary teaching programs but this, too, was ultimately resolved. The LCME, however, continued to wonder how a medical dean could "control" basic science departments which were also the administrative responsibility of other colleges.

Human Biology

In the earliest days of the college, the curriculum committee was chaired by a sociologist, who later served for several years as associate dean. The committee was composed of members of the preexisting basic and social science departments, with clinical representatives added as these disciplines were recruited. Our main consultant was Lester Evans, M.D., formerly a staff director of the Commonwealth Fund, who had been active in the landmark curricular change at Western Reserve. Liked and admired by all, he pushed us to consider what synthesis of available resources, in this huge university, could differentiate the scientific base for human medicine from that for other scientific or health-related programs. Struggling around this challenge, the committee developed the notion of human biology, defined broadly as the understanding of man as a biological and psychological unit, sharply responsive to ecological and sociological forces. This sequence, taught by faculty from relevant disciplines, would proceed alongside the disciplinary courses which the various departments had been developing for several years. In view of my pediatric background, the committee was influenced to put this learning sequence into the context of human development. One feature, for example, would be the physical examination of the newborn infant as the first-year students' first experience in "clinical relevance." (This tradition is maintained to this day.) While implementation of the human biology sequence was difficult, and while it did engender resentment on the part of some faculty members on the basis of interference with traditional departmental pedagogical prerogative, it served as the central feature of the curriculum for several years. While never overtly challenged by the LCME visiting teams, it seemed to have been viewed with skepticism.

Focal Problems

With the development of the Office of Medical Education Research and Development (OMERAD), faculty members, mostly in the departments of Medicine, Pediatrics, and Human Development, were recruited with a more sophisticated view of modern educational techniques and philosophy. It began to be felt that emphasis on process, rather than on content, might be more compatible with college goals, and that the core nature of Human Development might now be less viable. Capacity for life-long self-learning, and well-honed problem-solving ability as outcomes assumed high value with the curriculum planners. Furthermore, content learned in medical school should occur within the context of sharing with other students, rather than in the mode of grade-seeking competition. The result, partially derived from earlier experience at Western Reserve, was the "focal problem."[9] This was one of the pioneer ventures in problem-based learning via the small group discussion process. It involved the development of extensive and carefully prepared clinical paper cases including meticulously established reading lists and benchmarks for evaluation of student progress. Each student group of no more than twelve was led by a clinician and a basic biological or behavioral scientist. It featured student self-learning and limited the role of the preceptor to guidance and stimulation of discussion. It has recently been adopted by several distinguished medical schools. It is being actively supported as a concept by the AAMC, and has been the subject of an increasing spate of publications.[10] Administratively, an agency of the Deans Office was established with adequate budget and was staffed with skilled and informed personnel and a director who held both the M.D. and a Ph.D. in physiology. Over time, students in this program performed well in their evaluations. Furthermore, participation in the Focal Problem exercises was exciting for both students and faculty resource persons. In short, most of us felt that we had forged a major educational breakthrough.

This innovation, however, marked the beginning of our serious confrontations with the LCME. I remember well the first accreditation visit after the establishment of this program. The team's chair was known for his academic traditionalism; we could not help wondering why he had been chosen for this assignment. At the initial meeting, his first statement to me was: "Andy, we think your curriculum is Mickey Mouse." My rejoinder was to the effect that if he listened during the subsequent four days he might learn something. That, of course, occurred, and the team's final report, while accepting the focal problem as "perhaps" valid, suggested that we were too involved with such issues as sociology, and that we should turn our attention to the recruitment of a radiologist, and to a search for the "essential" university hospital. In all fairness, it must be acknowledged that the LCME never pressed us to eliminate the focal problem mode. We did feel, however, that it was their basic distrust of such pedagogy that fueled the escalation of their pressure on us to require National Boards, Part I before students entered their clinical years—and which finally led to our capitulation to this seemingly irresistible force.

The Community Hospital as the Base for Clinical Learning

On my recruitment, the president of Michigan State University, a land grant institution committed to the "people of Michigan," instructed me to develop a program that would be specifically oriented to the medical care needs of the state. An earlier survey of medical care in the state by an MSU sociologist had revealed a drastic shortage of young physicians in rural areas. We were not to attempt to compete ideologically with the great medical center at the University of Michigan, or with the Detroit-oriented Wayne State University. A strongly stated objective, then, was to work toward relieving the medical scarcity in the small towns and rural communities of Michigan. Indeed, it was this public commitment which helped to generate the ultimate legislative support necessary for success.

With the preclinical curriculum already oriented around problem solving and self-learning so important for the rural practitioner, we early on established community as both an area of research for our related social science departments, and as the locus of much of the students' clinical experiences. While the university planners had always assumed the ultimate presence on campus of a university hospital, and while our early years saw much effort in planning for one, we felt that community hospitals might well provide "real-life" settings for clinical clerkships with or without success in traditional medical-center development. Even the nature of the hospital we were contemplating would be combined with the university's student health service, and be intimately connected with our affiliated hospitals; its planning, therefore, was coordinated with the local hospital planning agency, with compromises made according to community bed needs.

Throughout this planning period we were developing programs for medical student clinical learning appropriate to the preclinical period of their education. This was not confined to Lansing (the location of the university), but also in other mid-Michigan cities such as Grand Rapids, Flint, Kalamazoo, and Saginaw. Appropriate hospital consortia in each community would ultimately develop, community physicians interested in teaching were further trained in community-based workshops on pedagogy provided by OMERAD, and a skilled nucleus of voluntary faculty emerged. The likelihood of acquiring a university hospital diminished as federal priorities changed during the 1960s and 1970s. With the first students entering their clinical years, we felt we were ready to launch a full four-year program with community hospitals as the sole locus for clinical clerkships in the core disciplines of medicine, including family practice.

Here we need to discuss the details of the intensive modifications required of the administration and fulltime faculty to make this work. They required specific budgetary and personnel allocations not customary in medical schools, such as extensive travel to the outlying communities by the East Lansing-based faculty, and creative solutions for administrative difficulties between normally independent hospitals needing to work together. The galaxy of potential problems was such that a permanent, fulltime, associate dean for community development was appointed, with assistant deans in residence in each of the five communities, including Lansing. Success has been striking, and one or more variants of this model have been utilized by other new schools without their own hospitals. A group of "community-based" medical schools has become a quasi-official subset of the AAMC's Council of Deans.

The LCME, however, has never been enthusiastic about this approach, significantly deviating as it does from a major tenet of the Flexner Report, and apparently flaunting the caveat that good medical education at the clinical level cannot occur in the absence of faculty control over a hospital's patient care. Medical schools in the community-based mode have, however, learned that control of patient care, while desirable, is not necessary if the educational objectives for students are clearly defined, if there is appropriate administrative supervision over the educational process, and if evaluation methodology measures student learning and progress according to the established objectives. Nonetheless, the absence of a university hospital has always been a hindrance to fully enthusiastic LCME approval. In fact, there appears to be a sort of unofficial and unwritten classification of medical schools, with some sort of "A" and "B" designation: "B" being those without hospitals, and not endowed with the same distinction as traditional academic medical centers.

The Upper Peninsula Program

The Upper Peninsula of Michigan, separated from the more densely populated Lower Peninsula, is generally rural with its copper mining industry in serious trouble. I became aware of the uniqueness and beauty of the Upper Peninsula early in my tenure at MSU when I worked on the draft of a Heart-Cancer-Stroke program with an academic surgeon who had retired there. The Upper Peninsula had long been a source of discomfiture for the governor and legislature, since its people, in view of its separation from the mainland by the Straits of Mackinac and because of the special nature of its cultural differences from the Lower Peninsula, had long felt separated, estranged, and politically, socially, and medically disenfranchised. While the area was sparsely populated with physicians, the city of Marquette supported a good hospital, Northern Michigan University, and an exceedingly competent and diversified medical society. It seemed clear that at some point our new medical school would find a way to work effectively in this area to provide a setting for our students to learn about a truly rural community, and would be politically helpful to the governor and the state legislature.

This opportunity came to pass with the development of a plan by Donald Weston, M.D., then associate dean and subsequently my successor at MSU, and James Thomas, a young faculty member. Their work, supported by the Rockefeller Foundation was written with a view toward increasing the effectiveness of medical education in third world countries or in rural America with a minimum of staff and expense.[11] The idea was that a university-based medical school with a core group of educational specialists (such as MSU's Office of Medical Education and Research and Development—OMERAD) and a small number of basic scientists and clinicians, supported by carefully developed focal problem programs and objectives, could sponsor the entire course of medical education in remote sites. This publication attracted the attention of the federal and state governments—the feds because of their interest in care in rural settings, and the state because of the apparent applicability of the scenario to the Upper Peninsula. In any case, intensive planning for such an endeavor was begun with federal help during the early 1970s. With Track II having been inaugurated in East Lansing as an alternate educational mode in which focal problems completely replaced lectures, intensive work in the development of paper cases to be used in the U.P. began. Detailed plans were made to locate a suitable facility in Escanaba to house both preclinical activities and outpatient facilities, and to recruit individuals to serve there as faculty. With the enthusiastic participation from both East Lansing-based faculty and from local practitioners, a small number of students committed to settle in the U.P. after graduation was recruited, and the program was launched. Students spent the first three months on the East Lansing campus where they experienced the same Phase I program provided to regular medical students. They then moved to the Upper Peninsula where their experience was divided between Escanaba for the first two years, and Marquette for most of the clinical years. Students learned well, as proved by their performance on examinations and, subsequently, as practicing physicians. A goodly number remained in the U.P. to practice.

The LCME, however, was horrified. We had, they said, proceeded with the program in the face of their threats of adverse accreditation action, and threatened such again unless the program were either discontinued or substantially modified. Program approval was not possible if medical students continued to learn their basic

125

sciences hundreds of miles from campus. Ultimately, full seven-year accreditation was achieved only after a compromise of principle, in which the preclinical years in the U.P. were discontinued and the program reduced to the status of just another locus for community-based clinical learning.

In my opinion, the LCME missed the chance to be a partner in an exciting educational experiment in which they could have jointly monitored evaluation instruments with a view to intellectually sound and imaginative exploration of ways in which medical education can really help with the difficult problem of rural medical care.

National Board Examinations

In the section entitled "Functions and Structure of a Medical School," under "Evaluation of Student Achievement," we read: "Each *provisionally accredited program must utilize methods for determining the quality of its program and the level of achievement of its students compared to national norms*" [italics mine]. It is to be noted that, when in the early days at Michigan State we were provisionally accredited as a two year program, we required students applying elsewhere for their clinical years to take Part I of the National Board examination. Later, however, when we were accredited as a four-year school, we dropped the National Board, Part I requirement, partly because we intended for basic science education to continue into the clinical years, and because we felt that the basic science hurdle at the end of the second year was counterproductive to the learning process. The LCME, however, continued to pressure us to adopt this measure. At the team visit which led our full seven-year accreditation, the National Board issue was the major area of discussion. It seemed clear that full accreditation depended upon our using these examinations at the end of the second year, with grades recorded and submitted periodically to the LCME.

While the school has survived these changes, and the basic curriculum has been retained, significant subjective alterations in student attitudes and values seem to have occurred. Current faculty find that a state of anxiety pervades preclinical students as they contemplate the stress of these examinations. While the generally eclectic nature of the curriculum persists, the feeling is that the original humanistic nature of the learning experience may have been significantly compromised.

Looking back on the accreditation process at Michigan State, I feel that during our formative years it was fair and constructive, especially when, largely for political reasons, the university administration was unreasonably pushing our timetable for admission of the first class. The authoritative voice of the LCME was used effectively in dealing with the state legislature. As we moved along, however, much of their impact was of questionable value. For example, in order to qualify for a Letter of Reasonable Assurance, we were required to have a written affiliation agreement with one of the major local hospitals (an item without which Harvard still gets along). This led to unnecessarily stormy meetings with the hospital staff, the development of an agreement which was almost immediately obsolete, and the beginning of a town-gown problem that is only now being resolved. Against my better judgment, this was forced on us by the LCME. As the curriculum developed, our innovations were often treated with disdain or outright hostility, in spite of our faculty's emerging preeminence in the field of educational research with the backing of the College of Education. The National Board compromise was the final price for seven-year accreditation. While the college survived this process, and while it remains a model for university-based medical schools effectively relating to the community, it was denied the privilege of full self-expression as a truly and importantly innovative educational effort.

Mercer University School of Medicine

State legislatures are not always satisfied with every aspect of the medical schools they sponsor. Many have emulated Ivy League models, have constructed huge medical centers, and have been successful in research productivity and the development of high-technology referral-type medicine. In terms of efforts to extend medical services to the poor within their own communities and rural parts of their states, however, they have often been found wanting. Their highest achievement in educational outcome is often the research-proficient specialist, and espousal of the family practice movement through the creation of relevant departments tends to occur only after legislative prodding. Some established state schools, such as Arkansas,[12] and a number of new schools have developed programs in rural health, a problem nationally recognized as deserving both educational and health planning attention.

Doubt remains, however, as to the viability of educating physicians specifically for careers in the socially deprived ambience of rural living. How many physicians and their spouses, for example, who are acculturated to the rich social and intellectual environment of the medical center, could comfortably exist in such settings? How could modern technology and communications serve to alleviate the problem? Such issues are not likely to assume high levels of priority among administrators and faculty of academic medical centers; they are usually relegated to subdivisions temporarily supported by program grants. The problem is so critical that it raises such difficult questions as the very viability of private practice as an effective deliverer of care among poor rural populations. It is difficult to see how a medical center that is based in research and high-technology medicine can fully and whole-heartedly lend support to such remotely relevant issues.

127

The Mercer University School of Medicine in Macon, Georgia, may be the first American medical school funded for and oriented toward relieving the medical shortage in the rural areas in its state. Mercer is a private, Baptist-supported institution with high academic standards. Its law school is recognized as one of the finest in the South. It is highly regarded and, with a reputation for responding to area and state needs, it has tended to be politically popular. The idea of a medical school developed in the late 1960s when the possibility of federal funding was suggested by a congressmen. I was invited, along with other deans and medical school officials, to a meeting in Atlanta in which the possibility of starting such a school was discussed with the university president and the first dean of the proposed school. It seemed to most of us that such a development was unlikely in view of the limited capacity of the home institution itself, which lacked any graduate programs in the sciences, but also because of questionable funding possibilities. About twelve years later, however, an attractive and functional building funded by a local bond issue and private contributions was constructed in Macon. The building included administrative and faculty office space, a considerable area designated for laboratory research, a fine medical library, large auditorium and classrooms, media and curriculum support services, and an outpatient center for health care. A dean who had served as an assistant dean at Michigan State was hired, a number of experienced faculty were recruited, and a curriculum was written under the aegis of an MSU graduate who had served as director of the Upper Peninsula program. Substantial annual funding had been acquired from state government, in view of the commitment of the university and its medical school to the relief of the shortage of primary care physicians in rural and other underserved areas of Georgia.

Mercer's new medical school became an immediate item of controversy. A medical school entirely devoted to rural primary care was unnecessary in the eyes of the state's two established medical schools which, of course, stood to lose a portion of their state appropriations if the new school really got underway. The original plans for the new school were indeed extraordinary. The strong emphasis on family practice proposed that the Department of Family and Community Medicine would be the only fulltime clinical department. The other usual specialties would be available from Macon and its large community hospital—the Medical Center of Central Georgia—which had fulltime specialists on staff. There was to be but one department of basic science encompassing all the traditional basic sciences except pathology. The basic science portions of the preclinical curriculum would be entirely in the mode of problem-based learning, and the introduction to clinical medicine would include closed-circuit television technology with simulated patients for interview training.

The commitment to primary care and rural medicine would begin with the admission process, which essentially would be limited to those Georgia applicants who clearly expressed a strong preference for such careers. While the definition of "primary care" included pediatrics, internal medicine, and obstetrics-gynecology, the main emphasis would be on family practice. The curriculum emphasized the school's basic objectives through a sequence entitled "Community Science," managed by the Department of Family and Community Medicine. It emphasized public health and featured two- to four-week preceptorships with rural practitioners during the first, second, and fourth years of medical school. These practitioners, recruited by the Family Practice Department, would become clinical faculty members. They would be involved in several workshops each year to plan and develop new aspects of the program. Part of each student's responsibility would be the writing of reports, community surveys, and the performance of public health-oriented research projects. By the end of this sequence, students would be well aware of the problems, issues, and opportunities that characterize rural medical practice.

Much of this rural-oriented program has survived the severe accreditation process to which Mercer was subjected, and is fully operational today. This is not to say that the program was lacking in challenges. I remember one visit during a "plenary" session with members of faculty and administration when the chair of the LCME committee described the problem-based-learning sequence as a "three-legged chicken." Reminded of my earlier experience at Michigan State University—the characterization of our curriculum there as "Mickey Mouse"—I felt impelled to deliver myself of comments in which I pointed out that such group process learning had been well tested at such schools as McMaster, Southern Illinois, and Michigan State, and that, by now, the chicken should have lost its third leg.

Nonetheless, the accreditation process at Mercer, although now apparently on the road to a successful conclusion, has been stressful in the extreme. While supportive in some ways, the first visit in 1982 foretold the problems to be encountered. From this site survey team's report we read: "Mercer is unique among recently developed schools of medicine appearing for first LCME evaluation in that it already has a completed, and occupied medical school building." The team was "delighted that Mercer has chosen the high road and has not settled for a trade school educational philosophy. We feel that there is an opportunity here to establish a model school for this type of curriculum and philosophy."[13] Thus, in this first visit, the team expressed basic support for an innovative curriculum relevant to the rural-primary care goals of the school. Criticisms, however, were clearly stated. Under the heading "Students," we find this caveat:

It is imperative that Mercer University School of Medicine attract and enroll well qualified students. The surveyors were deeply concerned with the qualifications of those students who have been identified for admission to the school of medicine. It is the viewpoint of the Survey Team that the present admissions process is unrealistic in that inadequate weighting has been directed to cognitive ability.

Concern about the problem-based curriculum was expressed, and this concern was clearly related to the dubious quality of students being recruited, for such a program imposes a "high degree of responsibility upon the student."

The team became agitated over the dominance of family medicine in the proposed clinical education program.

The surveyors recognize the fact that the MUSM has established as a goal that a high proportion of her graduates elect [to] practice primary care. Such a goal does not lessen the importance of the student receiving instruction in each of the major clinical disciplines. The survey team questions the absence of core clerkships in proposed curriculum phase D and E [third and fourth years]. We recommend that careful consideration be given to adding such core experiences in the major disciplines prior to subsequent LCME visits.

In accreditation jargon, this can only be interpreted as "do it or else!"

LCME concern about the program's capacity to succeed in view of some of the survey team's observations led to the following statement.

It is our view that all programs in medical education, whether experimental or traditional require careful measurement and evaluation both internally, and externally. Therefore, it is paramount that MUSM provide itself with an efficient way to assure that minimal national standards of medical education are being met. We recommend that as external measures of evaluation subtest examinations from Part I of the National Board of Medical Examiners be used at appropriate places in Phases A, B, and C.

Surprisingly, this LCME team did view "the organization of the traditional basic sciences into a division of biomedical science as appropriate for this school." This would require that a strong academic leader be recruited to assist the dean.

In any case, provisional accreditation for twenty-four students was awarded. The second visit came in December of the same year, followed by a limited visit in June. By this time, considerable progress was noted, with "the new junior year converted to more conventional clerkships with blocks in Internal Medicine, Pediatrics, Surgery, Obstetrics-Gynecology and combined comprehensive care clerkship (Family Medicine/Psychiatry)." Evidently, Parts I and II of the National Boards had been adopted, but "student records will contain notations regarding NBME only to the effect as to whether or not the student had passed Part I and Part II to satisfy the requirement for graduation." Again, the LCME awarded continuing provisional accreditation for a period of one year.

In February 1984, however, the university president was advised that in its February meeting the LCME had decided that MUSM "has not demonstrated sufficient progress in the development of its program ... that the program is not now in substantial compliance with the LCME's published accreditation standards, ... and that this constitutes grounds for placing the program on probation." While there were concerns about the length of the clerkship in internal medicine, the lack of progress in faculty recruitment, and the absence of a medical practice plan, the main problem was student performance on "shelf" National Board, Part I examinations (i.e., examinations given in previous years, but available for use in periodic testing of student progress). According to established procedures, the dean made an oral presentation to a LCME committee in which questions seem to have been satisfactorily answered. An April 1984 letter to the president lifted probation, and conferred provisional accreditation until October, 1984. A site visit in December 1984 found many improvements. Team members who visited some of the problem-based learning sessions were impressed with the Basic Medical Science program. They felt that the students were performing well, and that their level of knowledge was high. Once again, the "grave concern" that unqualified students were being accepted came up for discussion. Nonetheless, the site visitors felt that the admission process had improved greatly, and that the problem with NBME scores was resolving itself. The committee recommended lifting of probation. Our euphoria, however, was short-lived. In April 1985 the president received a letter from the LCME rejecting the team's report, and reaffirming one more year's probation. By that time, some of the accreditation difficulties had been blamed on the dean who, in May, was suddenly replaced. This was a traumatic event with accusations on both sides, and little explanation given the medical school personnel by the central administration. Fortunately, the new dean was well qualified and intimately informed on university, medical school, and Georgia politics. The transition was smooth, with the dean's status now elevated to include the office of Provost for Medical Affairs. The school's precarious accreditation status, however, was clearly one of his major concerns as he presided over another site visit in November 1985. This visit went well, but the committee's recommendation to lift probation was again denied by the LCME. An April 1986 meeting of the dean and a committee of the LCME was followed by a letter from the LCME discontinuing probation and granting full accreditation through November 1, 1986. The final visit in this tortuous sequence came in March 1987, after which Mercer was finally awarded a three-year period of full accreditation. Students have performed adequately on National Boards, and good residencies—mostly in the primary-care specialties—are being attained by the majority of the four graduating classes. In my opinion, students are of high quality and are unusually enthusiastic about their educational experience.

Since the last accreditation visit, the school has expanded its enrollment to 42 students per class and seems to be managing the increase successfully. The university, however, has recently suffered a considerable financial crisis. While this has not seriously affected the medical school, whose budget is specifically and separately identified, considerable anxiety has permeated the institution, where there have been cuts and salary reductions. The next accreditation visit, therefore, could be difficult, although the school's remarkable success should impress the visiting team favorably. As was our experience at Michigan State, the recurrent stresses of accreditation visits will continue for a number of years after the initial favorable LCME decision.

A review and critique of this process at Mercer reveals both the difficulties and ambiguities encountered by the LCME in unusual situations, and the stresses it imposes on institutions that are attempting to change critical aspects of medical education. As in Michigan, Georgia's expressed need was for a major alteration in the ratio of urban-oriented specialists to rural-oriented primary-care physicians, with a measurable increase in the number of doctors in such areas of medical shortage. The demonstrated lack of success by traditionally organized schools with standard curricula to accomplish such goals suggested the need for alternative administrative, staffing, and curricular arrangements. "Bandaid" curricular addenda seemed to be inadequate, and truly substantive innovations were required. A school so staffed and organized, therefore, might well differ significantly from the image of a medical school portrayed by the "Structure and Function" document. It would certainly be radically different from the modern academic medical center.

So far as the Mercer problem-oriented curriculum is concerned, the LCME would seem to have made considerable progress since the earlier characterization of the Michigan State venture into this mode as "Mickey Mouse." Although some ambivalence was still evident (as in the "three-legged chicken" discussion), there was never any LCME-directed effort to dissuade Mercer from this methodology. There was, furthermore, recognition that such a curriculum, as well as the single department of basic sciences, seemed appropriate to Mercer's declared institutional goals. The LCME was undoubtedly correct in its concern about the quality of the first medical class, and accurate in its assessment of the need for highly intelligent students to perform well in a self-learning mode. Subsequent classes have been of "better" quality, examination scores have improved, and the application pool is adequate.

The capacity of the LCME to support a valid risk was severely tested by a clinical program that downplayed clerkships in the traditional "core" disciplines. This the LCME found intolerable, and an ultimatum was issued to the effect that failure to institute such experiences might jeopardize accreditation. It seems to me that they missed an opportunity to help the school find ways to incorporate medical, surgical, psychiatric, obstetrical-gynecological and pediatric objectives into a family practice clerkship. With consultants from these core specialties in valid simulations of real-life family medical practice, the dominance of the primary care activity could have been preserved and enriched. Now, of course, excellent specialty clerkships occupy most of the third year, resulting in the usual surfeit of career options that dilute the degree to which the primary care objectives of the school are ultimately attained.

Finally, it is difficult for me to find rationale for stresses imposed by the imposition of probation. The adversarial relationship between the school and the LCME is far more destructive at all levels than can be justified by any accreditational progress it may stimulate.

Medicine is a favorite media topic. Front page headlines and prominent television coverage is assured with any major alteration in the status quo of hospitals or medical schools. The decision by a university to undertake medical education as a new venture almost always becomes a politically turbulent event. Opposition from other medical schools in the region usually takes the form of denying need for the new school, deploring projected costs, and inevitably asserting its general intellectual and professional inadequacies. Except possibly for local media outlets, the press is usually hostile. On my first trip to Lansing after my February 1964 appointment as dean at Michigan State, I was treated to an 11 o'clock television news diatribe on the effrontery of Michigan State to even contemplate such an irresponsible adventure into medical education delivered by the president of the University of Michigan in a speech to his alumni. This sort of thing is frequent during the first few years of a new school's history when the road for administration and faculty is inevitably uphill. Accreditation snags can be anticipated; the more innovative the plans, the more likely the snags. Real setbacks at the hand of the LCME intensify problems in such issues as legislative help, recruitment of faculty, fund raising, and attracting promising students. This is particularly ironic when, as in Mercer's case, part of the reason for probation was lagging faculty recruitment and a seemingly inadequate pool of qualified student applicants. For example, my own recruitment to Mercer came after a couple of consultation visits with the dean, who then learned of my interest in retiring to one of Georgia's Golden Isles where we had discussed the desirability of establishing a base for elective experiences in rural medicine. I had accepted a parttime position as assistant dean and was getting ready to move when I was visited in my

133

MSU office by my successor bearing the news of Mercer's probation, and wondering whether I might want to change my plans as a result. The gossip tom-toms had been working, and the news had spread like wildfire. Mercer's new kind of educational program assumed great public importance in Georgia. Graduates of established schools were quick to express skepticism about both the rural-practice goals and about the problem-based curriculum. The probationary status was widely known. In other words, while probation may have stimulated the medical school to correct some of its deficiencies, one can wonder about the wisdom of allowing such a damaging decision to become public knowledge. It seems to me that such adverse action as probation is really unnecessary in the face of the LCME's power, exercised quietly, with the threat of nonaccreditation as the main incentive for intensified university effort. At MSU, compromises and program modifications similar to those at Mercer had been exacted without the use of probation as a weapon.

While the medical school accreditation process officially stems from the LCME's document "Functions and Structure of a Medical School," it is clear that feelings, attitudes, and experiences of LCME members inevitably bear some influence on decisions. Since the majority of academic faculty and deans are products of traditional institutions, it is entirely understandable and perhaps prudent for the committee to be cautious about new educational or administrative departures. The staffs of the two parent organizations—the AMA and the AAMC—who maintain records, attend meetings, and provide continuity from year to year also can wield considerable influence. This was particularly true during most of the fifteen- to twenty-year period during which Michigan State, Mercer, and most of the other post-World War II schools developed. During that period, the AAMC Liaison Committee-related staff position fell to an unusually assertive, well-informed and traditional academic physician who quickly came to wield unusual power. He was exceedingly literate, at times humorous, and thoroughly convinced of the validity of the standard criteria of quality in medical education. Many deans perceived him to have become the czar of accreditation whose favor it was wise to cultivate and whose enmity was lethal. He seemed to dominate the process, and he strongly believed that there could be no justification for significant alteration of the academic medical center model. He appeared to reject any deviation from the traditional for specific purposes, such as emphasizing primary care. Community-based clinical experiences, especially during the first two years, were not welcome. He seemed dedicated to the unassailability of his interpretations of the "Functions and Structure" document—with whose writing he had been intimately connected. In a 1978 conference at Michigan State on "Medical Education since 1960"[14] there was free time for discussion as well as structured group participation. Deans from some of the new schools informally expressed resentment and frustration with the way in which various new programs and innovations in their schools were being treated by the LCME. In a group that was set up to encourage free discussion of these problems with him, not one dean, including myself, felt sufficiently comfortable in his presence to express these feelings of resentment or to ask questions which might have been helpful in clearing the air. In any case, it seems clear that during the period from about 1966 to 1984 accreditation served the purpose of guaranteeing adequate training of physicians graduating from new schools, but inhibited some worthwhile educational and administrative initiatives, and may well have retarded our profession's leadership in seeking out new arrangements and paradigms in American health care.

With the recent election of a new AAMC president, this accreditation position has been filled by another; a similar change has occurred at the AMA where, at this writing, an academician with many years' experience in medical school deanships is about to be installed as president. With the new AAMC president publicly espousing substantial change in medical education, and with the new AMA president proclaiming in pre-inauguration statements the importance of increasing accessibility of the American health care system, one can hope for a new era of more understanding and flexible medical school accreditation.

I have used my experiences in two new medical schools to appraise critically the accreditation process. My sole experience in an established university medical school was at Stanford in the early 1960s where an important new curriculum had been put into effect,[15] the result of five years of intensive planning, with strong emphasis on some of Western Reserve's innovations, and a considerable investment in behavioral science. During this period the school's administration had been equally active in the recruitment of distinguished faculty in such fields as genetics and biochemistry. The impact of these outstanding scientists was soon successful in opposing some features of the new curriculum, and the ambience of the institution began to resemble a research institute more than a school devoted to educational innovation. With its Nobel Prize-winning basic scientists, a superb and productive department of radiology, and a physical plant of great beauty, it had the potential to become one of the world's great medical centers. The LCME visit was, of course, generally favorable, but a number of recommendations for modest alterations were made. I well remember a meeting in the dean's office of the school's executive committee, in which the site visitors' report was discussed and found generally unworthy of compliance, with the comment that the visitors, mostly from state universities, just could not understand the complex issues being considered at a distinguished private institution such as Stanford.

I have participated in a number of site visits to established schools. Unless there was a financial emergency or administrative problem, we rarely had serious suggestions for the president and dean, nor were our recommendations ever overruled by the LCME itself. Indeed, since the "Functions and Structure of a Medical School" document is, in fact, derived from the model of the established academic medical center and usually reflects fairly precisely the image of the school being accredited, there is but little problem nor, at least in my experience, has LCME action resulted in impetus for significant change.

SUMMARY AND CONCLUSIONS

In a sense, the history of medical school accreditation recapitulates that of the AAMC and AMA. One of the main reasons for establishing the AMA in 1849 was to fight quackery and to control medical education at a time of intense medical pluralism. This was the beginning of regular medicine's power which has become today's monolithic, effective, and politically significant national organization. The AAMC, formed somewhat later, emerged as an organization of medical schools oriented around the details of curriculum, standards for faculty recruitment, and the promotion of research activity within the schools. The AAMC, marching under the banner of the Flexner Report and of medical education as an integral part of the university, has often proclaimed its independence from the AMA. However, efforts to implement organizational modifications such as those recommended by the Coggeshall Report to stimulate closer university ties, have failed to reverse the powerful tendency of medical schools to maintain a large element of independence from the general academic community. They have always been active in the clinical practice of medicine, essentially under AMA guidelines; surgical specialists, therefore, tend to achieve higher incomes than pediatric or medical doctors, largely through medical practice plans with fees-for-service established either on an individual or departmental basis. With such activity increasing during the current period of financial stress for medical schools, this tendency can but intensify.

The partnership with the AMA in the formation of the LCME in 1942 as the official accrediting agency for medical education consummates the relationship with the establishment of a vitally influential power center. In some ways, the academic medical center, with its huge faculty-controlled hospital and research establishment from which are culled most LCME members, mimics the proprietary institution which, in part, was the very reason for the educational revolution of the early 1900s.

There is great power within the LCME, and its jurisdiction over medical school certification has often generated friction with the universities within which the medical schools are located. While recent attempts to resolve this issue have apparently succeeded, some residual tensions remain. When we presented our findings to university presidents at some of the final meetings of site visit teams in which I have participated, I have felt uncomfortable with our arrogance, and have been disappointed with the docile fashion in which university officers have accepted our reports and occasionally unpleasant recommendations.

Reference has been made to the legal status of the LCME vis-à-vis the antitrust laws of the United States. Promoted by organized medicine as the most appropriate locus for medical activity, the private medical practice is essentially an independent small business, subject to the jurisdiction of these legal constraints. Thus, initiatives such as communitywide fee-setting may in fact be illegal and may open practitioners who indulge in such activity—however beneficial to the community—to prosecution. Likewise, the LCME, especially in view of the role of the AMA in its makeup, turns out to be subject to antitrust scrutiny. The study cited in this chapter avers that the monolithic nature of medical practice extends to the behavior of medical schools, medical specialists, and hospitals as well. The accreditation process tends to discourage competition between schools by insisting on the maintenance of a single model of function and structure, with virtually identical end-products. Accreditation of institutions and programs, as well as certification of specialists, therefore, is under the aegis of various self-appointed groups within the profession. While not "illegal" in the usual sense of the word, under the Sherman Act there is apparently an element of illegality. It seems conceivable that significant changes in medical school accreditation policies could emerge as a result of such legal pressures.

Havighurst's article cited in this chapter suggests that antitrust principles would limit the jurisdiction of the LCME to a general concern for quality and educational outcomes, rather than to details of individual program, staffing, and research productivity. We have referred repeatedly to the fallacy of National Board Examinations as valid measures of the quality of students and graduates, and of the notion that NBME test scores are adequate instruments to assess the comparative educational effectiveness of medical schools. While tests of cognitive knowledge, taken in the lonely locus of the proctored examination hall, may be useful guides to one benchmark of teaching effectiveness, they cannot measure broad institutional goals nor the potential effectiveness of physicians. Nor do they encourage diversity of educational goals between institutions, an apparently desirable objective vis-à-vis antitrust law. Assessment of such diversity would need to be linked to institutional missions. For example, a school like Stanford, with a stated objective of becoming a major source of research-productive academic medical scientists, must ultimately be judged by some measurement of how effectively such objectives have been met. Mercer's ultimate success will surely be measured by its ability to relieve the shortage of rural physicians in Georgia. The sum of Michigan State's medical faculty and its Lansing-based graduates now comprise more than one-third of the city's medical community; Lansing now has the lowest hospitalization rate in Michigan. The same reduction in Detroit could force the closing of up to one-half of its hospitals.[16] While certainly not the only factor in this accomplishment, the nature of the MSU program and its emphasis on ambulatory care is credited with a significant contribution to this situation; such an outcome, while not predicted, should be considered in the overall evaluation of a community-oriented institution. A wide variation in institutional styles, curricula, and general ambience is necessary for the attainment of multiple and varied institutional objectives. Indeed, I am informed that the LCME is presently revising its procedures to include in its evaluation of educational programs the degree to which stated institutional mission statements are met. One can hope, therefore, that the current reliance on National Board scores as a major criterion of educational success would in time become a thing of the past.

Medical school accreditation, as implemented through the Liaison Committee on Medical Education, has done well in assuring the prevalence of well-trained physicians but, at the same time, has generally served to maintain the status quo as expressed in the modern academic medical center. While enthusiastically supporting the kind of progress and change reflecting the accomplishments of biomedical research, the process has had great difficulty in recognizing the validity of change in reflecting advances in the social sciences, educational research, or resulting from conscious efforts to meet community health needs.

It is encouraging once again to hear presidential speeches,[17] and to read statements from the new AAMC-LCME staff person[18] that vigorously support courageous change-oriented behavior in individual schools. Unless such admirable exhortations are backed up by comparable support from the accreditation sector, however, little will actually happen. It will be recalled that similar inspirational utterances from the AAMC executive director in the early 1960s were not extended to the cold reality of accreditation. Recent speeches and papers from the new AAMC leadership are encouraging, and change may be in the wind. However, without full involvement of the power structure, as represented in the AAMC by the Executive Council and in the AMA by the Council on Medical Education and Hospitals, little progress can be expected, since it is by these councils that LCME members are selected. It is in the accreditation process that change in individual medical schools will or will not be tolerated, encouraged, or constructively used in the best interests of all.

138

NOTES

1. *Accreditation: A Statement of Principles*, The Committee on Institutional Cooperation, 302 E. John Street, Suite 1705, Champaign, IL 61820, February 26, 1987.
2. Meeting at AMA Headquarters, June 1988. Included Drs. Richard Egan, Harry Jonas, DeWitt Baldwin, and Barbara Barzansky, Ph.D., assistant to Dr. Jonas. The meeting (that I requested and taped), was in the form of free discussion, with my questions generally guiding the subjects discussed.
3. For example, four articles in the *Journal of Medical Education* 31, no. 8 (1956): J. T. Wearn, "Background and Philosophy," 516–18; T. H. Ham, "Method of Development and Revision in a Program of Medical Education," 519–21; J. W. Patterson, "Interdepartmental and Departmental Teaching of Medicine and Biological Science in 4 Years," 521–29; and J. L. Caughey, Jr., Clinical Teaching During 4 Years," 530–34.
4. George Miller, *Teaching and Learning in Medical School* (Cambridge: Harvard University Press, Published for Commonwealth Fund, 1961).
5. *Functions and Structure of a Medical School*, Accreditation and the Liaison Committee on Medical Education; *Standards for Accreditation of Medical Education Programs Leading to the M.D. Degree*, Liaison Committee on Medical Education, 1985. Now in the fall of 1990, this document is again being revised.
6. Ibid., "Introduction," 1.
7. Clark C. Havighurst and Nancy M. P. King, "Private Credentialing of Health Care Personnel: An Antitrust Perspective," Part One *American Journal of Law and Medicine* 9, no. 2 (Summer 1982): 132–201; and Part Two *American Journal of Law and Medicine* 9, no. 3 (Fall 1983): 263–334.
8. Daniel C. Schwartz, Acting Director, Bureau of Competition, FTC. A letter to Edward Aguirre, U.S. Commissioner of Education, November 11, 1976. Also a statement of Schwartz before the Advisory Committee on Accreditation and Institutional Eligibility, U.S. Office of Education, March 24, 1977.
9. J. W. Jones and P. O. Ways, "Focal Problems: A Major Commitment to Problem-Based Small Group Learning," in *Medical Education Since 1960: Marching to a Different Drummer* (East Lansing: Michigan State University Foundation and W. K. Kellogg Foundation, 1979). See also P. O. Ways, G. Loftus, and J. W. Jones, "Focal Problem Teaching in Medical Education," *Journal of Medical Education* 48 (June 1973): 565–76.
10. See, for example, H. S. Barrows, *The Tutorial Process: Southern Illinois School of Medicine* (Springfield: Southern Illinois School of Medicine 1988).
11. W. D. Weston, J. B. Thomas, and M. R. McGarvey, *Community Based Medical Education and Integrated Modular System of Health Care in Education* (East Lansing: Michigan State University Continuing Education Service, Kellogg Center, 1970), through the courtesy of a grant from the Rockefeller Foundation.
12. T. A. Bruce and W. R. Norton, *Improving Rural Health: Initiatives of an Academic Medical Center*. Little Rock: Rose Publishing Co., 1984.
13. Summary and Recommendations of LCME site visit survey team, January 10–14, 1982. All quotations and references to the confidential material in LCME reports are with the permission of W. Douglas Skelton,

M.D., Provost for Medical Affairs and Dean, Mercer University School of Medicine.

14. A. D. Hunt and Lewis E. Weeks, eds., *Medical Education since 1960: Marching to a Different Drummer* (East Lansing: Michigan State University Foundation, 1979), with cooperation and support of the W. K. Kellogg Foundation.

15. L. M. Stowe, "The Stanford Plan: An Educational Continuum for Medicine," *Journal of Medical Education* 34, no. 11 (1959): 1059–69.

16. W. D. Weston, personal communication.

17. R. G. Petersdorf, "Three Easy Pieces," speech at AAMC 1989 annual meeting. An elegant statement, using the analogy of a fairly recent moving picture, of the need for change in medical education. Probably soon to be published in *Academic Medicine*.

18. Donald G. Kassebaum, "Editorial: Change in Medical Education: The Courage and Will To be Different," *Academic Medicine* 64, no. 8 (August 1989): 446–47.

6
Summary and Recommendations

In this narrative the development of modern American medical education, from the mid-nineteenth century, has been traced. A major purpose of the AMA's early focus on physician education was to strengthen the status of regular medicine at a time when medical practice was fragmented into numerous cults—some scientifically sound, others labeled "quackery" by traditionally educated physicians. At the same time, the idea of medical practice as an assortment of independent private ventures, licensed by state boards largely under the control of physicians themselves, became institutionalized as the normal way in which medical care was provided. Later in the century, along with the American industrial revolution and the resultant availability of wealth for higher education and medical research, European—especially German—standards of academic medical education became institutionalized here, with Johns Hopkins emerging as the model research university sponsoring a medical school. With the acceptance of financial help from the corporate establishment, largely from foundations, both medical practice and medical education became identified with political and social conservatism.

For many years universities such as Harvard, Pennsylvania, and Michigan had sponsored quality medical schools that were usually under the control of physicians. The existence of poorly equipped and educationally inadequate proprietary schools, however, remained an embarrassment to the AMA's Council on Medical Education and Hospitals, which moved to survey the existing institutions in order to elevate standards and to identify which schools should be closed. Included in the rationale for such a study was a general dissatisfaction with the social status of medicine, especially in view of the differences that had been observed in Germany. As a supposedly neutral agency, the Carnegie Foundation was enlisted to duplicate the AMA's study. This was accomplished by Abraham Flexner, whose classic document, the 1910 *Bulletin Number Four* propelled him into the role of super-ego for medical education—and powerful advocate of university-dominated medical education.

Flexner's advocacy of high academic standards has been interpreted as a banner under which the dominance of research and the rigidity of administrative and curricular form became essential to the maintenance of high quality. The academic medical center has grown to colossal stature, status, and influence. The AMA and AAMC have combined to form the Liaison Committee on Medical Education, and this body, as it accredits medical schools, has favored the form and function of the academic medical center as the educational norm, with efforts to deviate from this standard only reluctantly accepted.

With new leadership in the AAMC, in the staffing of both AAMC and AMA arms of the LCME, and in the AMA itself, there is evidence of renewed interest in the need for reform of curriculum and a greater tolerance for relevant administrative modifications. We have seen, however, that in the cases of two enthusiastically innovative new medical schools, the accreditation process inhibited major initiatives designed to modify effectively the educational process in the interest of relevance to problems in our medical care system.

Eli Ginsberg has written of his problems finding reasonable medical care in New York with its specialized scene, and concludes that the mere expansion of numbers of generalists will do little to solve the problem. The explosive growth of the uninsured population and the "widening spread in levels of health care received between white and black, between affluent and poor, and between inner city and suburban residents raise questions about our commitment to equity." He goes on to say that there is little to be expected from "any effort to increase the number and proportion of generalists in the absence of antecedent and concurrent transformation in the structure and functioning of academic health centers and the financing of medical care, as well as major, long-lasting changes in the delivery of health care."[1]

Fundamental change in most of the great academic medical centers, however, seems unlikely. Their tradition is too strong; their commitment to clinical research and high-technology care has been too ingrained into their very structure and financial success; and the governmentally imposed restrictions on use of research funds, and on the ways in which, for example, Medicare-financed hospitalizations are managed are among the forces that tend to perpetuate the present structure and function. Perhaps the best that can be hoped for is sponsorship by some medical centers of social medicine units to operate community-based programs and research in the provision of health services, and to maintain community-oriented programs in fields such as adolescent medicine, and the care of patients suffering from AIDS.

It is important, however, to remember the enormous contributions of the academic medical center to research and to health profession education at all levels, and to recognize its essential nature in the development of increasingly effective specialized care. It seems incumbent on the establishment that has created the academic medical center, however, to turn attention to the correction of the serious defects in the present system of American medical care.

Medical education, and the research and patient care delivered by medical school faculties, set the standards of excellence, style, and behavior of the nation's physicians. This dominance over the way in which medicine is practiced does not stop with graduation. Through universally available programs in continuing education—generally provided by medical school faculty under the sponsorship of county medical societies, community hospitals, medical specialty societies, professional journals, medical school departmental grand rounds, and weekly cable television programs—this influence lasts an entire professional lifetime. In general, it is true that our lifelong system of medical education is effective, and serves to develop and maintain a very high level of quality in physician performance that serves patients and communities well. While high-quality life-long education of physicians under these auspices is available, there is also a dark side. Many continuing education programs are commercially sponsored by pharmaceutical houses or equipment manufacturers on topics that are relevant to the product being promoted. (Under the sponsorship of a community hospital I have attended more than one CME lecture that was an unabashed drug commercial delivered by a competent medical school faculty member accompanied by a detail person with relevant leaflets and drug samples.) Furthermore, continuing medical education programs tailored for practicing physicians rarely seem to be concerned with problems in the delivery or economics of medical care. Rather, they deal with such issues as recent technical developments, or are restatements of ways to solve interesting diagnostic problems. Indeed, we have noted in chapter 4 how the system, based in the research-rich academic medical center, works best in maintaining the skills and competence of the highly specialized physician. In other words, CME tends not only to reinforce the status quo of medical practice, but also to further the disease-oriented specialization of today's medicine. My own experience as a client of the health care system illustrated the effectiveness of modern specialized medical care in a small to middle-sized community as it coped with my moderately serious condition. While the medical skill and hospital technology was the equal of that in the academic medical center, and the ultimate outcome was excellent, my post-operative course was complicated and stormy. In my opinion this was mostly due to two closely related factors: the total reliance for medical care on my extramurally office-based surgeon with routine daily physical examinations performed by nurses with limited skill and experience; and the administrative delegation of dietary responsibility to a nonmedical service department. Although this criticism in no way is intended to detract from the dedication, professional integrity, or medical, nursing, or administrative competence of the group who cared for me, it does, however, suggest weaknesses in the organization of community health care and implies the need for patient-oriented planning to achieve the best results in an increasingly technological age. It has implications not only for undergraduate and graduate medical education, but for nursing and hospital administration as well. This is not a limited problem. Recent national reports of unexpectedly high hospital mortality rates, whose causes are related to issues similar to those I have just mentioned, have serious implications for fundamental organizational arrangements. Attention needs to be paid, then, not only to increasing accessibility of medical care, but to certain critical planning and organizational details. These are clearly matters for the serious attention of organized medicine and medical education.

Ever since the failure of the Truman administration to pass the Wagner-Murray-Dingell Bill, many medical economists and other experts in the health care field have been predicting the failure of our medical care system, and urging radical change during the decade to follow. While some changes have occurred, such as federal reimbursement for disadvantaged populations, the emergence of prepaid group practices (HMOs), and the improved health benefit plans for employees and retirees developed by industrial, academic, and other employers, the basic "bottom line"—the profit motive for nearly all participants in the health care complex—has not been altered. Some of the best buys on the stock market are the offerings of pharmaceutical houses and producers of high-tech medical equipment. National hospital corporations are turning much of the hospital industry into a profit-making enterprise and, through management arrangements, are turning failing community hospitals into paying propositions. This is accomplished, in part, by increased efficiency, but also by increasing rates, lowering in-service education budgets, cutting back on staff, and diminishing the availability of hospital care to the poor and uninsured. Physician fees are increasing at a pace well beyond the national inflation rate. While the inordinately complex malpractice issue—with its attendant rise in liability premiums—can be faulted for some of the increased costs of doing business, the net income of physicians continues to escalate. Fees continue to be set according to what the physician thinks his services are worth, and what the traffic will bear. The impact of antitrust laws on efforts to avoid physician competition by establishing communitywide fee schedules has resulted in an increased tendency to make fee-setting a private matter. This trend has led one writer to describe American health care as a "cost-unconscious system."[2] Indeed, the cost of medical care seems to be among our major problems. While quality, communication, and other details of the physician-patient relationship are vital aspects of care, and are intimately related to the malpractice issue, cost remains the hurdle which must be addressed for our system to remain intact.

I have traced the emergence of American medicine as critical player in the medical-industrial complex, and have become convinced that physicians' education and acculturation are dominant in maintaining most aspects of the system: good, bad, and indifferent. The recent authorization by the AAMC of the GPEP Report, recent speeches by the new president, the retirement of its previous chief of accreditation, an apparently increased flexibility within the LCME, and the plethora of current articles on educational change suggest a new willingness to consider appropriate refashioning of some of the ways in which students learn the art and science of medicine.

I am not certain, however, that the intensity of the inertia resisting change is always recognized. I was recently invited as consultant to a traditional medical school in the Southeast whose dean had appointed a small faculty committee to study the possibility of floating an effort in problem-based-learning for the preclinical years. While the committee was well-informed and enthusiastic about the concept, a subsequent meeting with a group of department chairs revealed widespread hostility to the entire notion. Such pedagogy was labeled "inefficient," unscientific, wasteful of limited resources and, in general, inappropriate for a distinguished institution. I am certain that such feelings run rampant among most faculties, and that they take these attitudes with them as they develop AAMC and LCME policy. While the AAMC's new support of workshops to help institutions adopt such pedagogical change could be helpful, my experience leads me to doubt that they will be successful without some previous preparation of faculties for major change not only in curriculum but also in relevant administrative modifications and budgetary reallocations.

Of equal or even greater importance than pedagogical technique to real modification of physician practice, attitude, and societal relevance is faculty role-modeling during the clinical years and in residency training as students learn about patient care through involvement in the process. With medical fees a major problem today, faculty income could have high priority. A recent issue of the *Chronicle of Higher Education*,[3] quoting from IRS records, indicated the frequency of inflated medical faculty incomes, often at levels higher than those of university presidents. That such is the case is hardly surprising in view of the competition with the private sector in recruitment and retention of faculty. However, the extreme nature of the discrepancy is, in a few instances, shocking—namely, academically connected surgeons with annual incomes exceeding $1 million. Such extravagant benefits from the right choice of career are not lost on medical students, who may well be going deeply into debt just to stay in school. In the 1986 Mercer graduation speech, Ferrol Sams,[4] a well-known Georgia physician and writer, spoke of the "obscenity" of such incomes by physicians, and implored the graduates not to be "obscene." (It is my understanding that it was not received with total enthusiasm by all of the physicians present.) In any case, the issue of physician income must be addressed with leadership from the academic community.

The problem of cost containment is being addressed in many medical schools, usually through such exercises as decision analysis, and making students aware of the costs of commonly ordered laboratory and therapeutic procedures. However, unless students see their professors putting such considerations into practice as they care for their patients in the medical center or clinic and in the context of that pinnacle of academic performance, departmental grand rounds, such learning can come to naught.

The current movement toward the increased use of ambulatory services for student and residency training is certainly a step in the right direction. Here again, one must be certain that such ambulatory teaching is done not only by faculty identified as "primary care physicians," such as those in departments of family practice, or by selected junior members of traditional academic departments, but also by senior and research-oriented faculty who really listen to patients, demonstrate effective collaboration with nursing and other health professions, espouse such modalities as home health care and hospice, and who put into practice principles of medical ethics learned by students earlier in their medical school experience. Finally, such criteria of capacity to practice in a patient-oriented fashion should be included in the relevant evaluation of student performance.

In chapter 5, I emphasized the critical role of accreditation and the power of the LCME in institutionalizing the quality, style, and scope of medical education. The imagination, dedication, and skills of medical faculties, the willingness of administration to channel these energies in innovative ways, and the quality of initiatives displayed by students are among those attributes constituting the necessary condition for thoughtful change in medical education. The sufficient condition for the success of such change is the support and encouragement of the AAMC and AMA, and its implementation through the process of accreditation. I have shown how the accreditation process has in the past worked mostly to inhibit movement of medical education away from traditional form, content, and style, and have also noted how the present makeup of the LCME and its AMA and AAMC staffs could presage changes in attitude and decision making.

The LCME could, then, be in a position to recognize the need for diversity in the functions and structure of medical schools, and to establish criteria of excellence for those that deviate from the traditional pattern. It might even become a protective umbrella under which institutions could undertake seemingly outrageous programs with appropriate central guidance, so that accreditation site visits would be transformed from exercises in hostility to collegial consideration of goals, objectives, evidence of progress, and of the necessary scholarly activity upon which the innovative program was based. Quality, although perhaps occasionally redefined, would be maintained.

A major part of the challenge to the educational system is not only to recognize its responsibility for leadership as the nation struggles with its health and medical problems, but also to recognize the immense effort entailed in assuming such leadership. At a recent Council of Teaching Hospitals' meeting, health economist Rashi Fein urged physicians, especially COTH members, to become politically active in states that are attempting to implement new health care programs. Citing the federal deficit as a retardant to nationally developed programs, he was urging health professionals to become active at state and local levels.[5] In another *Weekly Report*, however, we find the following. In describing a meeting of the AAMC-Academic Health Centers (AHC) Forum, where a number of medical issues were discussed, one topic was "the inadequate access to health care for a substantial part of the nation's population: it was apparent that the necessary leadership at the national level was lacking, although the group could not determine which sector of society had the responsibility or the influence to assume this role."[6] It would have been reassuring had some mention been made of a possible role for the AAMC. In my estimation, the content of the guidelines for accreditation used by the LCME is far too limited to encompass expanded visions of the scope of medical education. The manual mentions several times that individual medical practice is the activity toward which medical school and residency training is directed. At one point, for example, under "Educational Program for the M.D. Degree," it is stated that "the curriculum of the program leading to the M.D. degree must be designed to provide a general professional education, recognizing that, this alone, is insufficient to prepare a graduate for *independent, unsupervised* practice.[7] The idea that the ultimate goal of medical education is the production of a host of independent and unsupervised practitioners is clearly not the intent of the authors of the "Functions and Structure" document. They themselves are personally aware of the multiple options available to medical graduates, such as the intensely structured and supervised practice within a fulltime department of medicine, of research and administrative careers, and of opportunities for leadership in the nation's social and political systems.

It would seem most likely, therefore, that the capacity to practice medicine independently and without supervision is seen by the AAMC and AMA leadership as a necessary condition for a physician and as a measure of specialty qualifications. It seems to me, however, that this focus on trade-like skills trivializes not only the nobility and scope of our great profession, but also the social responsibilities of the LCME and its sponsors. It tends to support the widespread public impression of the self-serving nature of much of the activities of American physicians, and to reenforce suspicions that the primary consideration of organized medicine and its educational establishment is its own social and financial well-being. (I bitterly recall a dinner party shortly after our arrival at Michigan State given in our honor by an academic economist, whose opening statement as we sat down at the table was: "The medical profession is motivated chiefly by greed!")

It is time to come to terms with official and public recognition that, while the private-enterprise locus of medical care, with its dependence on the research and educational activities of academe and the engineering and pharmaceutical productivity of the industrial sector, has given the United States a spectacularly successful system for the paying public, its weaknesses are being given wider recognition. I am writing this on the last day of the 1980s; today's newspaper stresses the potentially devastating effect of AIDS on the health-care system, with 14.5 million AIDS-related deaths predicted by the year 2002, the skewing of these deaths toward the black and Hispanic populations, the tragic impact of drugs, and the threat of the impact of an overturning of *Rowe* vs *Wade* on the innercity population explosion. In the business section, we find the headline: "More businesses shifting burden of health premiums to employees." The article states that in 1984, 53 percent of employers' health plans reimbursed 100 percent of hospital costs; today but 29 percent. The converse follows, of course, with a marked increase in the magnitude of deductibles. A pie graph as to why employees do not have health insurance shows multiple reasons, with "can't afford it" the largest fraction, at 35 percent. While the Social Security fund is growing, with surpluses expected for the next thirty years, the president's new budget projects some decrease in funding for Medicare.[8] These concerns for the future of America's health and its ability to cope with the problems and costs, and the potential impact of such developments upon the very structure of society seem clearly to be weighing on the minds of the lay public.

A few days ago, the *AAMC Weekly Report* arrived. The president's holiday message thanked the AAMC constituency and staff for a productive and rewarding year, and named some of its challenges:

> ... in such issues as the use of fetal tissue in medical research, conflict of interest, the use of animals in research and changes in Medicare funding policies. We have followed closely the federal government's actions on appropriations for such crucial budget components as medical research, NIH, the VA, Medicare payments for hospital and physician services, and student loans.
>
> The year ahead promises to hold new challenges and accomplishments in academic medicine and research. As leaders in medical education, we must continue to work together to resolve the pressing problems we face.[9]

The need to cope with the housekeeping and maintenance details of medical schools still seems to take precedence over the ability or desire of the AAMC to respond to the paramount issues facing the public and practicing physicians in matters of health and medical care. It is time that the AAMC power structure—and that of the AMA as well—face up to the fact that, contrary to the earlier dream of Gates and the pioneers of modern medical education, biomedical research alone is an insufficient basis for the education of all physicians for all of modern society. It should recognize the essentially conservative nature of this paradigm and its analogy to the "trickle down" notion of conservative political doctrine. The practice style resulting from such a base, while often technically superb, is wont to be extravagant. Without consideration of humanistic and ethical considerations it can be brutal and inhumane.

I fear collapse of the system within the next decade or so unless significant changes come to pass. While I am at a loss to define the precise nature of the changes that will be needed, I am certain that the AAMC, in collaboration with the AMA, is essential to guiding the process which will be required to ascertain what should be done in education, research, organizational planning, political action, and collaboration with all levels of government. An unusual degree of recognition of the need for modifications in their life-styles, sources of income, and the ways in which they relate to governmental and other nonprofessional agencies will be needed by physicians in order for appropriate alterations in the system to occur. It would seem unlikely for such adaptability to result from any means other than intense involvement of the major national medical organizations.

During the mid-1970s I was privileged to participate in several management seminars sponsored by the AAMC and implemented by members of the faculty of the Massachusetts Institute of Technology. While MIT's focus was on the corporate sector of private enterprise, a main emphasis in these sessions was the importance for companies to keep abreast of social change, and to do all in their power to foresee accurately what might happen in the future. Dubbed "strategic planning," and implemented by specifically designated institutional "think tanks" unfettered by policy or administrative constraints, they explore predictable turns of social events, and feed options for institutional response to management for appropriate decision making. They felt strongly that such a process was essential for a corporation's continued success.

The analogy with health and medicine seems clear. Our continued success as a huge and profitable member of the private enterprise system is conditional on the way we can adapt to society. Whether we can accomplish control of our costs, whether we can deliver the best ethical, patient-oriented care to our paying public and, perhaps above all, whether we can truly collaborate with government and other social agencies in guaranteeing that the benefits of modern medicine be extended to those currently unable to avail themselves of this remarkable system, are some of the questions which must soon be answered.

What course, then, is open to medical schools, the AAMC, the AMA, and the LCME to help smooth the way to physician participation, even leadership, in the national political and social effort to rectify the shortcomings of our present medical care system? I am not discussing the political, economic, and organizational ventures which will emerge, and in which organized medicine will participate in one way or another. In accord with the emphasis within this entire monograph, I am limiting my suggestions to those related to medical education and the academic medical center. I do this as one who has loved his academic career, has deeply admired his AAMC and AMA colleagues, disagreements notwithstanding, and with unaccustomed humility. Such suggestions might include the following.

1. The next rewrite of the "Functions and Structure of a Medical School" should recognize that the "independent unsupervised practitioner" is but the beginning of the definition of a physician. A more complete description should include such features as demonstrated scientific ability, humility, literacy, leadership capacity, broad understanding of our health system's strengths and weaknesses, demonstrated capacity to ethically analyze a medical moral dilemma, recognition of the limits of private practice, and a broad understanding of the issues concerning delivery of medical care to disadvantaged populations. It is perfectly possible to develop instruments to evaluate these characteristics.

The self-study materials distributed to medical schools prior to accreditation visits should include evidence of administrative and curricular arrangements to insure the students' achievement of such educational and experiential objectives. The site-visit teams should make special efforts to explore the degree to which such goals and objectives have been met, and should include positive and negative findings appropriately in their reports and recommendations for LCME action.

2. Strategic planning is an activity that could well be adopted by individual medical schools. Issues confronted by such planning bodies, while continuing to be concerned with the health of biomedical research, would be heavily weighted toward social problems in medical care and how the schools could respond most effectively to them. I feel that the AAMC—probably jointly with the AMA, and involving government and industry as well, possibly within the context of the LCME, and in some sort of harmony with similar activity in the individual schools—should also engage in a national version of strategic planning. Progress in this activity should be a main feature of plenary sessions in the AAMC annual meetings. Such presentations could fit in well with the political and idealistically resounding talks that characterize these effective and often stimulating sessions.

150

3. The *Weekly Report*, the AAMC's organ of regular communication with its medical schools, should place much more emphasis on the relevance of AAMC activity to the issues of delivery of medical care, reports on what individual schools are doing in this area, and even suggestions as to how individual schools might be more effectively involved in such issues.

4. The AAMC and AMA should attempt to influence continuing medical education programs to widen their spectrums of offerings to include difficulties, dilemmas, and progress within the field of medical care.

5. From what most of what the nation's media tells us, one might suppose that academic medical centers are totally occupied with such procedures as organ transplantation and open heart surgery. One must assume that institutional public relations departments emphasize these dramatic scientific and surgical feats in the interest of fund-raising and national prestige. The fact is that virtually every academic medical center, while fundamentally organized around bench research and tertiary care, has at least one program or administrative division demonstrating or conducting socially-oriented research in some aspect of community health.

I have mentioned the initiative in rural health at Arkansas. An exciting program on urban health in the Bronx is supported by the Montefiore Medical Center/Albert Einstein College of Medicine.[10] While continuing to be thrilled by examples of spectacular successes in academic medical centers, much of the American public is probably weary of tales of surgical tours-de-force and semi-martyrdom of near-folk heroes on the altars of scientific and technical progress. Evidence that an important element of the academic establishment also cares about the health of disadvantaged people at home might come as welcome and even surprising information.

6. Finally, the AMA needs to be involved at many levels, but particularly through its influence over programming by its constituent state and county medical societies. This organization now appears to be aware that the health of the private practice of medicine is threatened by its escalating costs and its incapacity per se to serve disadvantaged populations. Without the intervention of society—usually in the form of government—to provide the funds needed for individuals and families to obtain essential elements of medical care from practicing physicians, these populations are eliminated as beneficiaries of the system. The threat of the AIDS epidemic could provide added impetus for organized medicine to abandon its traditional fear and dislike of governmental "intervention" in the conduct of its affairs. In any case, governmental intervention to facilitate the continued validity of private practice is surely far less threatening than, for example, total federalization of physicians. I was recently impressed by an exceedingly thoughtful discussion in a local medical society on this sort of issue. The widespread occurrence of such discussions would greatly help prac-

ticing physicians to become leaders in the modification of relevant aspects of medical practice.

It seems safe to predict a continuation of fundamentally conservative politics in the United States, especially in view of the striking decline in the power and extent of centralized socialistic governments abroad. This should buy time for several years, during which significant resurgence of political pressure for drastic metamorphosis of our medical system is unlikely. This period should also provide the opportunity, through leadership from the medical profession itself, to generate sufficient change to insure that our system, with its great research tradition, magnificent educational record, and highly successful diffusion of successes to the community settings, can proceed to serve the public well. Resulting from the change, health, generally mediated through medicine, could become uniformly affordable, and readily available to our entire society.

NOTES

1. Eli Ginsberg, Ph.D., "Do We Need More Generalists?" *Academic Medicine* 64, no. 9 (1989): 495–97.
2. Alain Endhoven, "A Cost Unconscious System," *New York Times*, July 1989.
3. "Many Medical Professors at Private Research Universities Earn More than Presidents," *Chronicle of Higher Education* 36, no. 3 (1989).
4. Ferrol Sams, commencement speech, Mercer University, June 1, 1986.
5. *AAMC Weekly Report* 4, no. 19 (1990).
6. *AAMC Weekly Report* 4, no. 22 (1990).
7. "Functions and Structure of a Medical School," Liaison Committee on Medical Education, 1985, p. 13, italics mine.
8. *Florida Times-Union* (Jacksonville), December 31, 1989.
9. *AAMC Weekly Report* 3, no. 45 (December 21, 1989).
10. V. W. Sidel, Apollo Asklepios, and Zeus, "Health Community, and Government," address at the graduation of the class of 1989, Mercer University School of Medicine, June 1989; also by Sidel, "Public Health in International Perspective: From Helping Victims to Blaming to Organizing Them," *Canadian Journal of Medicine* July 1979, 70: 234–239.

Bibliography

AAMC Institutional Profile System Ranking Report. Run on 11/06/87. Request 2015: Research Expenditures.

AAMC Weekly Report 3, no. 42 (1989); 3, no. 45 (1989); 4, no. 19 (1990); 4, no. 22 (1990).

AAMC. *Washington D.C. Weekly Report* 3, no. 42, (1989).

Association of American Medical Colleges. "Academic Medicine Faces the Future." *1988–89 Annual Report.*

————"American Medical Education: Institutions, Programs, and Issues." AAMC staff report, Robert F. Jones, Director of Institutional Studies, Division of Planning and Development, 1989.

Bambara, A. J., and A. D. Hunt, Jr. "Specialist Plus, Not Versus, Family Physician: A Setting Conducive to Effective Postgraduate Education." *Postgraduate Medicine* 20 (1956): 305–9.

Barrows, H. S. *The Tutorial Process: Southern Illinois School of Medicine.* Springfield: Southern Illinois School of Medicine 1988.

Baughman, B. B. "The Beginning of the Medical School of the University of Kentucky; the Political and Scientific Background; Louisville, 1979." *Journal of the Kentucky Medical Association* 77 (1979): 525–28.

Beauchamp, T. L., and J. F. Childress. *Principles of Biomedical Ethics.* New York: Oxford University Press, 1989;

Benjamin, Martin, and Joy Curtis. *Ethics in Nursing.* London: Oxford University Press, 1981.

Berliner, Howard. "New Light on the Flexner Report: Notes on the AMA-Carnegie Foundation Background." *Bulletin of History of Medicine* 51 (1977): 603–9.

Bevan, Arthur D. "Minutes, Council on Medical Education." *JAMA* 44, no. 18 (1905): 1470–75; and *JAMA* 48, no. 20 (1907): 1701–7.

Bierring, Walter L. "Early Licensing and Subsequent Decadence: 1650–1875." *Federation Bulletin* 43, no. 4 (1956): chapt. 1.

————"Medical Licensure after Forty Years." *Federation Bulletin* 43, no. 4 (1956).

Bonner, Thomas N. *American Doctors and German Universities: A Chapter in International Intellectual Relations, 1870–1914.* Lincoln: University of Nebraska Press, 1963.

Brody, Howard. "Transparency: Informed Consent in Primary Care." *Hastings Center Report* 19, no. 5 (1989): 5–9.

Brown, E. R. *Rockefeller Medicine Men.* Berkeley: University of California Press, 1979.

Bruce, Thomas. *Education for Rural Medicine.* Fayetteville: University of Arkansas Press, 1984.

Bush, Vannevar. *Science, the Endless Frontier: A Report to the President on a Program for Postwar Scientific Research*, July, 1945. Reprinted, Washington, D.C.: National Science Foundation, 1960.

Caughey, J. L., Jr. "Clinical Teaching During 4 Years." *Journal of Medical Education* 31, no. 8 (1956): 530–34.

Chapman, Carleton. "The Flexner Report by Abraham Flexner." *Daedalus* 103 (1974): 105–17.

Chesney, A. M. *The Johns Hopkins Hospital and The Johns Hopkins School of Medicine: A Chronicle*, vol. 1. Baltimore: The Johns Hopkins University Press, 1943.

Coggeshall Lowell. *Planning for Medical Progress through Education.* Evanston, Ill.: Association of American Medical Colleges, 1965.

Committee on Institutional Cooperation. *Accreditation: A Statement of Principles*, February 26, 1987.

Cooper, John A. D. "The Association of American Medical Colleges: Looking Ahead from the First Hundred Years." *Journal of Medical Education* 52 (1977): 11–19.

———"Physicians for the Twenty-First Century, The GPEP Report." Washington, D.C.: Association of American Medical Colleges, 1984.

Corner, George W. *A History of the Rockefeller Institute, 1901–1953, Origins and Growth.* New York: Rockefeller Institute Press, 1964.

"Council on Medical Education of the AMA, the Chairman, Dr. A. D. Bevan, Presiding." *JAMA* 58, no. 20 (1907): 1701–7.

Culver, C. M., et al. "Basic Curricular Goals in Medical Ethics." *N.E.J.M.* 312 (1985): 253–56.

Darley, Ward. "The Association of American Medical Colleges: Its Objectives and Program." *Journal of Medical Education* 34, no. 8 (1959): 814–18.

———"AAMC Milestones in Raising the Standards of Medical Education." *Journal of Medical Education* 40, no. 4 (1965): 321–27.

Editorial. "The Core Content of Family Medicine, a Report of the Committee on Requirements for Certification." *GP* 34 (1966): 225.

"Ecology of the Medical Student. Report of the Fifth Teaching Institute, AAMC, Atlantic City, N.J., October 15–19, 1957." *Journal of Medical Education* 33, no. 10 (1958).

Endhoven, Alain. "A Cost Unconscious System." *New York Times*, July 1989.

Englehardt, H. Tristram, Jr., and Daniel Callahan. *Science, Ethics and Medicine.* Hastings on Hudson, N.Y.: Institute of Society, Ethics and the Life Sciences, 1976.

"Evaluation in the Continuum of Medical Education." Report of the Committee on Goals and Priorities of the National Board of Medical Examiners, Philadelphia, 1973.

Fickenger, K. M. "Medical Education and Rural Health Care: Responsibilities and Opportunities." Presentation at AAMC Annual Meeting, November 1989.

Fleming, Donald. *William H. Welch and the Rise of Modern Medicine.* Baltimore: The Johns Hopkins University Press, 1954, 1987.

Fletcher, Joseph. *Morals and Medicine.* Boston: Beacon Press, 1954.

Flexner, Abraham. *Medical Education in the United States and Canada; A Report to the Carnegie Foundation for the Advancement of Teaching*, Bulletin Number Four. Boston: D. P. Updike, The Merrymount Press, Boston, 1910.

———*Medical Education, A Comparative Study.* New York: MacMillan Company, 1925.

154

————"I Remember." The Autobiography of Abraham Flexner. New York: Simon and Schuster, 1940.

Florida Times-Union (Jacksonville), December 14, 1989; December 31, 1989.

Fox, Daniel. "Recent Marxist Interpretations of the History of Medicine in the United States," Clio Medica 16 (1982): 225.

Functions and Structure of a Medical School. Accreditation and the Liaison Committee on Medical Education, 1985.

Galetti, P. M. "Brown University; Division of Biological and Medical Sciences." In The Case Histories of Ten New Medical Schools, edited by V. W. Lippard and E. F. Purcell. New York: The Josiah Macy Fr., Foundation, 1972.

Gates, Frederick. "Memoirs of Frederick T. Gates." American Heritage 6, no. 3 (1955): 73–74.

Geiger, H. J. "The Neighborhood Health Center: Education of Faculty in Preventive Medicine." Archives of Environmental Health 140 (1967): 912–16.

Geyman, John P. Family Practice: Foundation of Changing Health Care, 2d ed. Norwalk, Conn.: Appleton-Century-Crofts, 1985.

Ginsberg, Eli. "Do We Need More Generalists?" Academic Medicine 64, no. 9 (1989): 495–97.

Graduate Education of Physicians. Report of the Citizen's Commission on Graduate Medical Education (Millis Commission). Chicago: American Medical Association, 1966.

Ham, T. H. "Method of Development and Revision in a Program of Medical Education." Journal of Medical Education 31, no. 8 (1956): 519–21.

Harrell, G. T. "The Pennsylvania State University, The Milton S. Hershey Medical Center." In The Case Histories of Ten New Medical Schools, edited by V. W. Lippard and E. F. Purcell. New York: The Josiah Macy Fr., Foundation, 1972.

Harvey, A. McGehee, and Susan L. Abrams. For the Welfare of Mankind: The Commonwealth Fund and American Medicine. Baltimore: The Johns Hopkins University Press, 1986.

Havighurst, Clark C., and Nancy M. P. King. "Private Credentialing of Health Care Personnel: An Antitrust Perspective," Part One. American Journal of Law and Medicine 9, no. 2 (Summer 1982): 132–201; and Part Two American Journal of Law and Medicine 9, no. 3 (Fall 1983): 263–334.

Higher Education and the Nation's Health. Policies for Medical and Dental Education. A special report and recommendations by the Carnegie Commission on Higher Education. New York: McGraw-Hill Book Company, 1970.

Hudson, Robert, M.D. "Flexner and the 1990s." A symposium in Chicago, Illinois, June 10–11, 1986.

Hunt, A. D., Jr. "At a Rural Hospital" (part of a symposium on the hospitalized child). Children 3 (1956): 90.

————"Michigan State University, College of Human Medicine." In The Case Histories of Ten New Medical Schools, edited by V. W. Lippard and E. F. Purcell. New York: The Josiah Macy Fr., Foundation, 1972.

————"The Impact of Abraham Flexner upon Teaching in American Medical Schools." A symposium entitled "Flexner and the 1990s" in Chicago, June 10–11, 1986.

Hunt, A. D., Jr., and Lewis E. Weeks, eds. Medical Education since 1960: Marching to a Different Drummer. East Lansing: Michigan State University Foundation and W. K. Kellogg Foundation, 1979.

"Implementing GPEP." Eighth Annual Conference for Generalists in Medical Education, November 8 and 9, 1987, Embassy Row Hotel, Washington, D.C.

Jones, J. W., and P. O. Ways. "Focal Problems: A Major Commitment to Problem-Based Small Group Learning." In *Medical Education Since 1960: Marching to a Different Drummer*. East Lansing: Michigan State University Foundation and W. K. Kellogg Foundation, 1979.

Jonsen, A. P. "Leadership in Meeting Ethical Challenges." *Journal of Medical Education* 62, no. 2 (1987): 95–99.

Kassebaum, Donald G. "Editorial: Change in Medical Education: The Courage and Will To be Different." *Academic Medicine* 64, no. 8 (August 1989): 446–47.

Kant, Immanuel. *Groundwork of The Metaphysic of Morals*. Translated by H. J. Paton. New York: Harper and Row, 1964.

Kunitz, Stephen. "Professionalism and Social Control in the Progressive Era: The Case of the Flexner Report." *Social Problems* 22: 16–27

Liaison Committee on Medical Education. *Functions and Structure of a Medical School. Standards for Accreditation of Medical Education Programs Leading to the M.D. Degree* (1985).

Lippard, Vernon W. *A Half Century of American Medical Education, 1920–1970*. New York: Macy Foundation, 1974.

Ludmerer, Kenneth M. *Learning to Heal: The Development of American Medical Education*. New York: Basic Books, Inc., 1985.

MacIntyre, Alasdair. *A Short History of Ethics*. New York: Macmillan, 1966.

"Many Medical Professors at Private Research Universities Earn More than Presidents." *Chronicle of Higher Education* 36, no. 3 (1989).

Marston, R. Q., et al. "Regional Medical Programs: A Progress Report." *American Journal of Public Health* 58 (1968): 726–30.

"Medical Education and Medical Care." Report of the Eighth Teaching Institute, AAMC, Hollywood Beach, Florida, November 1–3, 1960. *Journal of Medical Education* 36, no. 12 (1961).

"Medical Licensure after Forty Years." *Federation Bulletin* 43, no. 4 (1956).

Meeting the Challenge of Family Practice. Report of the Ad Hoc Committee on Education for Family Practice of the Council on Medical Education. Chicago: American Medical Association, 1966.

"Memoirs of Frederick T. Gates." American Heritage 6, no. 3 (1955): 73–74.

Mill, John Stuart. *Utilitarianism*. Indianapolis: Bobbs-Merrill, 1957.

Miller, George, S. Abrahamson, I. S. Cohen, H. P. Graser, R. S. Harnack, and A. Land. *Teaching and Learning in Medical School*. Cambridge: Harvard University Press, Commonwealth Fund, 1961.

The New York Times, February 28, 1988, E-5.

"Objectives of Undergraduate Medical Education." *Journal of Medical Education* 28, no. 3 (1953): 57–59.

Odoroff, M. E. "Measuring Progress of Regional Medical Programs." *American Journal of Public Health* 58 (1968): 726–30.

Parran, Thomas. *The Aims of the Public Health Service*. Smithsonian Institution Annual Report, 1937 (Washington, D.C.: Government Printing Office, 1938.

Patterson, J. W. "Interdepartmental and Departmental Teaching of Medicine and Biological Science in 4 Years." *Journal of Medical Education* 31, no. 8 (1956): 521–29.

Pellegrino, E. D. "State University of New York at Stony Brook Health Sciences Center." In *The Case Histories of Ten New Medical Schools.* Edited by V. W. Lippard and E. F. Purcell. New York: The Josiah Macy Fr., Foundation, 1972.

Petersdorf, R. G. "Three Easy Pieces." Speech at AAMC 1989 annual meeting. *Academic Medicine*

"Physicians for the Twenty-First Century: The GPEP Report." Report of the Panel on the General Professional Education of the Physician and the College Preparation for Medicine. Washington, D.C.: Association of American Medical Colleges, 1984.

———"Commentary on the GPEP Report." Adopted by the Executive Council of the Association of American Medical Colleges, September 12, 1985.

Progress and Problems in Medical and Dental Education: Federal Support Versus Federal Control. Report of the Carnegie Council on Policy Studies in Higher Education. San Francisco: Jossey-Bass, 1976.

Rawls, John *A Theory of Justice.* Cambridge: Harvard University Press, 1971.

Report of the First Institute on Clinical Teaching, Swampscott, Mass., October 7 to 11, 1958." *Association of American Medical Colleges,* 1959.

Report of the Second Institute on Clinical Teaching, Report of the Seventh Institute, AAMC, Chicago, Ill., October 27–31, 1959, *Journal of Medical Education* 36, no. 4 (1961).

Research Activity of Full-Time Faculty in Departments of Medicine. Washington, D.C.: APM and AAMC, 1987.

Reverby, Susan, and David Rosner, eds. *Health Care in America: Essays in Social History.* Philadelphia: Temple University Press, 1979, chapt. 10.

Riska, Elianne. "Social Reform and Reform in Medical Education." In *Medical Education Since 1960: Marching to a Different Drummer.* Edited by A. D. Hunt and L. E. Weeks. East Lansing: Michigan State University Foundation, 1979.

———*Power, Politics and Health: Forces Shaping American Medicine.* Helsinki: Finnish Society of Sciences and Letters, 1985.

Roosevelt, F. D. "Letter on the Office of Scientific Research and Development." *Science* 100 (1944): 542.

Rosner, David. *A Once Charitable Enterprise: Hospitals and Health Care in Brooklyn and New York, 1885–1912.* Cambridge: Cambridge University Press, 1982.

Rothstein, William G. *American Medical Schools and the Practice of Medicine, a History.* New York: Oxford University Press, 1987.

Sams, Ferrol. Commencement speech, Mercer University, June 1, 1986.

Schnauss, D. C. "Comprehensive Health Planning: A Boon or a Bane?" *Hospital Programs* 48 (1967): 63–67.

Schofield, J. R. *New and Expanded Medical Schools, Mid-Century to the 1980s.* San Francisco: Jossey-Bass Publishers, 1984.

Shorter, Edward. *The Health Century.* New York: Doubleday, 1987.

Shyrock, Richard H. *American Medical Research.* New York: The Commonwealth Fund, 1947.

———*Medical Licensing in America, 1650–1965.* Baltimore: The Johns Hopkins University Press, 1967.

Sidel, V. W., Apollo Asklepios, and Zeus. "Health Community, and Government." Address at the graduation of the class of 1989, Mercer University School of Medicine, June 1989.

157

Skelton, W. Douglas. "Primary Care Education and Service: The Role of Medical Schools." Speech delivered at the AAMC Council of Deans, Spring Meeting, Sanibel Harbour Resort, Florida, April 1990.

Smiley, Dean F. "History of the Association of American Medical Colleges." *Journal of Medical Education* 32, no. 7 (1957): 512–25.

Smith, Page. *America Enters the World*, vol. 7. New York: McGraw-Hill Book Company, 1985.

Starr, Paul. *The Social Transformation of American Medicine*. New York: Basic Books, Inc., 1982.

Stowe, L. M. "The Stanford Plan: An Educational Continuum for Medicine." *Journal of Medical Education* 34, no. 11 (1959): 1059–69.

Strickland, Stephen P. *Politics, Science, and Dread Disease: A Short History of United States Medical Research Policy*. Cambridge: Harvard University Press, 1972.

"Teaching of Anatomy and Anthropology in Medical Education, AAMC, Swampscott, Mass., October 18–22, 1955." *Journal of Medical Education* 31, no. 10 (1956) (in two parts);

"Teaching of Pathology, Microbiology, Immunology, Genetics, Report of the Second Teaching Institute, October 10–15, 1954." Part 2, *Journal of Medical Education* 30, no. 9 (1955): 91.

"Teaching of Physiology, Biochemistry, Pharmacology; Report of the First Teaching Institute, AAMC, Atlantic City, October 19–23, 1953." *Journal of Medical Education* 29, no. 7 (1964) (in two parts).

Trussel R. E. *Hunterdon Medical Center: The Story of One Approach to Rural Medical Care*. Cambridge: Harvard University Press, 1956.

U.S. Department of Health and Human Services. *1987 NIH Almanac*. NIH Publication no. 87–5, September 1987.

U.S. Congress, Senate. Committee on Military Affairs. *Report from the Subcommittee on War Mobilization on Wartime Research and Development*, 1940–44, pt. 1: vii.

Veatch, Robert M. *Case Studies in Medical Ethics*. Cambridge: Harvard University Press, 1977.

Watson, J. D. "The Human Genome Project: Past, Present, and Future." *Science* 248 (1990): 44–49.

Ways, P. O., G. Loftus, and J. M. Jones. "Focal Problem Teaching in Medical Education." *Journal of Medical Education* 48 (1973): 565–76.

Wearn, J. T., et al. "Reports on Experiments in Medical Education." *Journal of Medical Education* 31 (1956): 515–65.

———"Background and Philosophy." *Journal of Medical Education* 31, no. 8 (1956): 516–18.

Weston, W. D., J. B. Thomas, and M. R. McGarvey. *Community Based Medical Education and Integrated Modular System of Health Care in Education*. East Lansing: Michigan State University Continuing Education Service, Kellogg Center, 1970.

Wyngaarden, James B. "A Century of Science for Health." *Clinical Research* (1988).

Index

Medical Education, Accreditation, and the Nation's Health

Production Editor: Julie L. Loehr
Design: Lynne A. Brown
Copy Editor: Jo Grandstaff
Indexed by: Ellen Link
Text composed by: Delmas Typesetting, Inc.
in 10 pt. Century Schoolbook

Printed by McNaughton & Gunn
on 55# Glatfelter B16

Smyth sewn and cased in Roxite B Linen
with black matt stamp